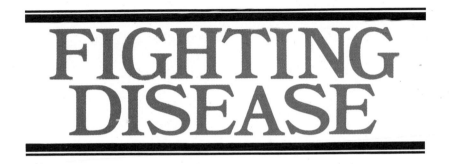

FIGHTING DISEASE

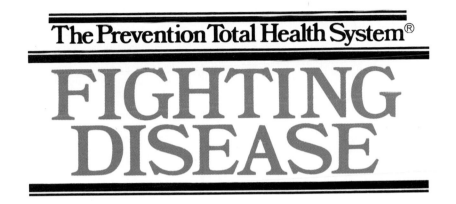

The Prevention Total Health System®

FIGHTING DISEASE

by the Editors of
Prevention® Magazine

 Rodale Press, Emmaus, Pennsylvania

Library of Congress Cataloging in Publication Data

Main entry under title:

Fighting disease.

(The Prevention total health system)
Includes bibliographical references and
index.   1. Health.   2. Medicine, Popular.
I. Prevention (Emmaus, Pa.) II. Series
RA776.F514 1984   613   84-6971

ISBN 0-87857-487-5 hardcover
6 8 10 9 7 5   hardcover

NOTICE

This book is intended as a reference volume only, not as a medical manual or guide to self-treatment. If you suspect that you have a medical problem, we urge you to seek competent medical help. Keep in mind that nutritional and health needs vary from person to person, depending on age, sex, health status and total diet. The information here is intended to help you make informed decisions about your health, not as a substitute for any treatment that may have been prescribed by your doctor.

The Prevention Total Health System®
Series Editors: William Gottlieb, Mark Bricklin
Fighting Disease Editor: Carol Keough
Writers: Sharon Faelten (Chapters 1, 6, 11); William D.
     Ehrhart, Laura Rosetree (Chapter 2); Susan
     DeMark (Chapters 3, 9); Marian Wolbers (Chapter
     4) with William D. Ehrhart, Susan DeMark;
     Stephen Williams (Chapters 5, 8); Mark O'Brien
     (Chapter 7) with Jan Bresnick; Martha Capwell,
     Stephen Williams (Chapter 10).
Research Chief: Carol Baldwin
Assistant Research Chief, Prevention Health Books:
     Christy Kohler
Researchers: Holly Clemson, Susan Nastasee, Carol
     Pribulka, Joann Williams, Barbara Balas, Martha
     Capwell, Sue Ann Gursky, Carol Matthews, Pam
     Mohr, Anne Oplinger, David Palmer, Carole Rapp,
     Camille Romig, Nancy Smerkanich, Pam Uhl,
     Susan Zarrow
Copy Coordinator: Joann Williams
Series Art Director: Jerry O'Brien
Art Production Manager: Jane C. Knutila
Designers: Lynn Foulk, Alison Lee
Illustrators: Susan M. Blubaugh, Joe Lertola,
     Anita Lovitt, Donna Ruff
Associate Designer: John Pepper
Director of Photography: T. L. Gettings
Photo Editor: Margaret Skrovanek
Photographic Stylists: Renee R. Grimes, Kay Seng
     Lichthardt, Scott Schmidt, J. C. Vera
Photo Librarian: Shirley S. Smith
Staff Photographers: Angelo M. Caggiano, Carl Doney,
     T. L. Gettings, Mitchell T. Mandel, Alison Miksch,
     Margaret Skrovanek, Christie C. Tito
Copy Editor: Jane Sherman
Production Manager: Jacob V. Lichty
Production Coordinator: Barbara A. Herman
Composite Typesetter: Brenda J. Kline
Production Administrator: Eileen F. Bauder
Office Personnel: Diana M. Gottshall, Susan Lagler,
     Carol Petrakovich, Cindy Harig, Marge Kresley

Rodale Books, Inc.
Publisher: Richard M. Huttner
Senior Managing Editor: William H. Hylton
Copy Manager: Ann Snyder
Art Director: Karen A. Schell
Director of Marketing: Pat Corpora
Business Manager: Ellen J. Greene
Continuity Marketing Manager: John Taylor

Rodale Press, Inc.
Chairman of the Board: Robert Rodale
President: Robert Teufel
Executive Vice President: Marshall Ackerman
Group Vice Presidents: Sanford Beldon
                                       Mark Bricklin
Senior Vice President: John Haberern
Vice Presidents: John Griffin
                        Richard M. Huttner
                        James C. McCullagh
                        David Widenmyer
Secretary: Anna Rodale

Contents

Preface   vii

Chapter 1: The Heart of Good Health   1
> When you rejuvenate your heart and arteries,
> you rejuvenate your life. Here's the plan.

Chapter 2: Help for Troubled Breathing   19
> Smart choices in lifestyle are your surest
> defense against breathing disorders.

Chapter 3: Freeing the Joints   33
> Our bones, joints and spine can retain
> the fluid grace of youth.

Chapter 4: Facing the Cancer Challenge   53
> Simple changes in lifestyle and diet may well
> be our best weapons against the disease.

Chapter 5: Upper Digestive Problems   69
> Take the heat out of heartburn and ulcers.
> Using diet, combat gallstones and kidney stones.

Chapter 6: Calming a Stressed Intestine   87
> Sorting the truth from the myths of
> digestive problems can spare you a lot of
> pain and indignity.

Chapter 7: Diabetes: The Sugar Disease   103
> Insulin isn't the *whole* answer. Along with
> medication, don't overlook the benefits
> of fiber-rich foods and exercise.

Chapter 8: Diet Rules the Skin's Health   113
> What you eat plays a big role in preventing skin
> diseases like psoriasis, shingles and acne.

Chapter 9: Caring for the Health of Women   123
> Prevention and knowledge have revolutionized
> women's health care.

Chapter 10: The Mind and the Senses   135
> A sound body and a sound mind are one. If diet
> heals the body, then it also can heal the mind.

Chapter 11: Freedom from Addictions   155
> Not "bad habits," addictions are real illnesses
> that can be treated and often cured.

Source Notes   164

Credits   165

Index   165

Self-Care Has Come of Age—Again!

Some 30 or 40 years ago, there was general belief that "scientific medicine" would in short order obliterate just about all disease. Optimism continued to mount as new antibiotics and tranquilizers were discovered, new surgical procedures devised and space age diagnostic techniques perfected. For a while it seemed that if we could all live just a few more years, new discoveries might make us immune to death itself.

Looking back, we can see that the party mood began to sour about 10 or 15 years ago. More and more people suspected that medicine's voyage of discovery had degenerated into a mere joyride of doctoring.

Antibiotics and tranquilizers were prescribed—and swallowed—like Good & Plenty's. X rays were ordered for trivial reasons. Surgery rates climbed like the bull stock market, and medical bills followed.

It was not just an innocent burst of enthusiasm. Real harm was done. Drugs, we all learned, sometimes had a tail called "side effects." Needless X rays were thought to promote cancer. Many operations, we learned, were ineffective or unnecessary or both.

But that's only half of the new perspective. The other half has this to say: Even when done correctly, even when done with care and compassion, the medical approach to disease is incomplete. Wonderful, yes. But not quite the whole answer.

What it ignores is the dimension of natural healing: strengthening the body's immune system through nutritional and other natural means; physical therapies; stress reduction; diet improvement; and lifestyle change. To ignore these factors is to forgo, perhaps, a much more conservative, perhaps even more effective treatment. And even when extensive medical intervention *is* required, we now know, the battle against disease cannot be won by medicine alone. Unless the body has sufficient vitality to recover from the trauma of intervention, then reestablish a state of health that will prevent the return of disease, medicine may be for naught.

Some people reacting against what they see as overdoctoring have rejected the technological approach almost completely. They have returned, in effect, to the 19th century, relying on herbs, untested diets and unscientific procedures to treat all illness.

But there is no need to reject *all* of modern medicine because of its occasional excesses. Nor is total rejection very smart. Today, we are in the unique position of being able to take advantage of the best technological medical care *and* the best natural healing techniques.

By using both approaches, as dictated by good sense, we can literally enjoy the best of two worlds.

The information and ideas in this book are therefore meant to complement the guidance you receive from your physician, not to replace it. Doctors today are becoming more aware of the alternative and natural approaches to health and may be perfectly willing to discuss them with a patient who expresses interest.

Many readers will find this volume of The Prevention Total Health System® to be of special interest. It may well open a new world of health possibilities to you. Read it, learn and, together with your doctor, arrive at a well-rounded plan of health-restoring therapy.

Executive Editor, **Prevention**® Magazine

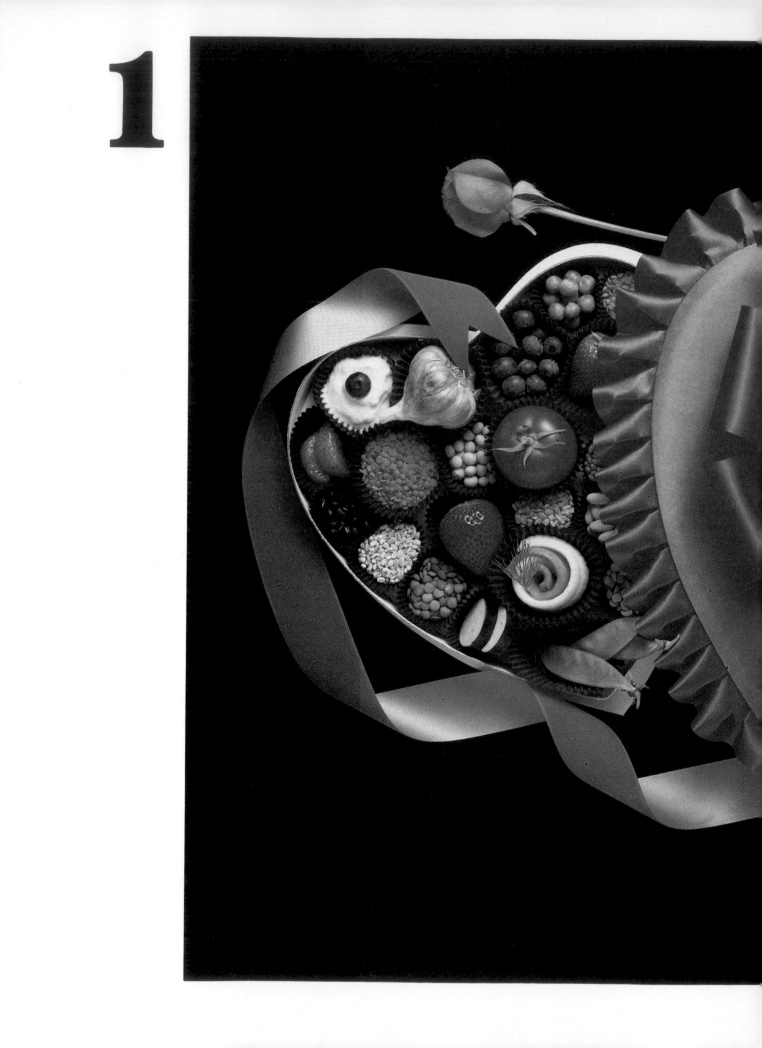

1

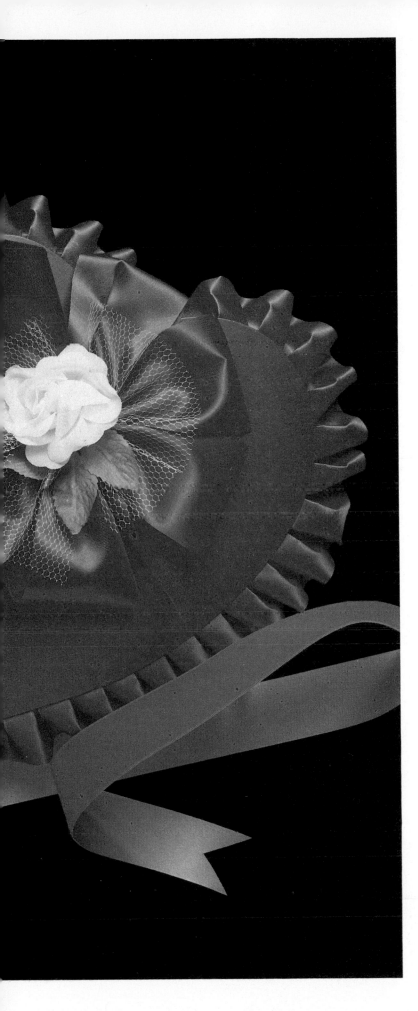

The Heart of Good Health

When you rejuvenate your heart and arteries, you rejuvenate your life. Here's the plan.

If a nuclear power plant accidentally blew up and wiped out a million Americans, the entire country—the entire world, for that matter—would panic. Yet a million Americans die every year from another type of disaster—the personal disaster of heart disease. In fact, this disease is the number one killer in the U.S., accounting for half of all deaths, including accidental deaths of all types. Consider this variety of common heart and circulatory problems:

- Hypertension (high blood pressure), in which the contraction of small arteries causes constant high-throttled pumping of blood that may wear out the heart and arteries;
- Atherosclerosis, which occurs when a buildup of artery sludge blocks the lifeline of blood;
- Stroke, caused by a major blockage of blood flow to the brain;
- Thrombophlebitis, a condition marked by clots in the deep veins, usually in the legs; and
- Angina, disabling, recurrent pain that can be a prelude to a heart attack.

The alarm sounds loudest for people who have a family history of heart disease; those who overeat and underexercise; those who smoke; or for people who have diabetes or high levels of cholesterol (a type of fat) in their blood. Any one or any combination of these risk factors can put you in the danger zone. But the good news is that you can do a great deal to prevent heart disease, or lessen the severity of an existing condition.

HYPERTENSION: THE SILENT KILLER

The low, persistent moan of a foghorn was the only sound in the sleeping city. Harry walked briskly between the deserted factories, his footsteps clicking on the glistening cobblestones. He sensed that he was in danger, although frequent, darting looks over his shoulder revealed the street was empty.

Harry reached his car and quickly climbed in, locking the doors. But no locks could protect him from the silent killer stalking him.

The killer, you see, was within him. It was hypertension (high blood pressure). And it stalks 37 million Americans a year. The killer favors blacks over whites and older people over young, although plenty of non-blacks and even teenagers are affected.

Hypertension is truly a senseless crime against the body, because it can be easily overpowered, once detected. But first let's start by finding out just what makes this killer "tick."

Normally, blood courses through your arteries and veins with the greatest of ease. In fact, any number of quite normal things can force the heart to pump harder than usual, and thus elevate blood pressure—things like getting angry or barely avoiding a traffic accident. But when blood pressure continues to overtax the arteries day after day, month after month, it severely batters them, along with harming the organs these blood vessels serve. This damage happens quite silently, without severe pain or other warning. Then, suddenly, the damage becomes all too apparent.

Often, the problem is compounded by the presence of fatty plaque in the battered arteries, a condition that can lead to a heart attack. Or blood can backwash into the lungs, causing congestive heart failure. Or high-throttled blood pressure can rupture small blood vessels in the brain (triggering a stroke), in the eyes (causing blindness) or in the kidneys (causing kidney failure). If untreated, 50 percent of all people with high blood pressure will die of heart disease, 33 percent will die of stroke and 10 to 15 percent will die of kidney failure.

If you have high blood pressure, here's what to do. Begin by swearing off the salt shaker and cutting down on high-sodium foods. Sodium has been indicted as a prime suspect in high blood pressure on the basis of three kinds of circumstantial evidence. First, people who live in societies whose members eat very little salt rarely have high blood pressure, while people who live in societies where there is high salt intake (like the U.S.) frequently have high blood pressure. Second, animals with a genetic tendency toward high blood pressure ultimately develop this condition if they eat more salt than the body actually requires. This fact strongly implies that the same thing happens to people who, because their parents have hypertension, are predisposed to the disease.

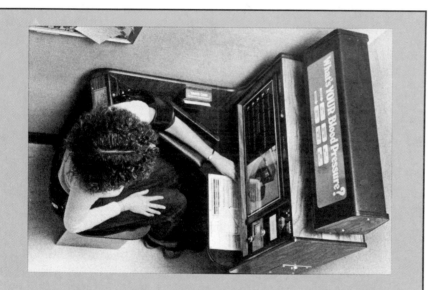

What Those Numbers Mean

Blood pressure is so easy to measure that you can do it yourself. Blood pressure monitors show up in airport lounges and under Christmas trees. Just strap on the cuff, inflate it, and listen to your pulse through a stethoscope pressed against an artery. At first no sounds are heard as the cuff begins to deflate. The first sound you hear will be a tapping noise. This is the pulse at peak artery pressure, or systolic pressure. When the cuff deflates further, the sounds disappear as the artery pressure reaches the lowest point, or diastolic pressure.

Systolic and diastolic pressure register as numbers on the attached meter. A normal ratio of systolic to diastolic pressure is 120 over 80 (though somewhat lower is perfectly healthy). Anything higher than 140 over 90 is considered high blood pressure.

Third, and even more convincing, studies have found that people with high blood pressure have more sodium in the walls of their blood vessels than do people with normal blood pressure.

If eating *more* sodium raises blood pressure, eating *less* should lower it. And to a great degree, cutting down on sodium does help enormously. One study reported that among 16 patients given only dietary advice—including the dictum to cut down on salt—12 lowered their blood pressure significantly after two months of cutting back their intake by 40 percent.

If you think that salt-free living is easier said than done, consider this: Rinsing food is a simple, practical and economical way to help reduce sodium intake. In an experiment at Duke University Medical Center in North Carolina, chemists drained canned green beans and rinsed them under tap water for 1 minute. The sodium content of the beans dropped by 41 percent. Rinsing canned tuna for 1 minute cut sodium content by up to 79 percent.

Cutting salt intake, however, is only one step in the counterassault against high blood pressure. Doctors have found that sodium has a symbiotic relationship with another mineral, potassium. The more potassium you eat, the less sodium is able to raise blood pressure.

In fact, potassium may be the long-sought key to why vegetarians, as a rule, have lower blood pressure than nonvegetarians. A study was done of vegetarians who ate no meat, no fish, no more than three eggs per week, and very little milk and few milk products. They *did* eat plenty of fruit, vegetables, and nuts—all rich sources of potassium. Sodium intake was roughly equal in both groups. What wasn't equal was blood pressure—the vegetarians' was lower. The researchers concluded that the vegetarians, by consuming so much potassium, blunted sodium's effect on blood pressure.

You don't have to become a vegetarian to experience the benefits of potassium. In fact, you need take only two simple steps: Eat foods rich in this mineral and cook them in a way that preserves as much potassium as possible. Steaming is one such method. For example, potatoes are considered an excellent source of potassium. But Swedish researchers discovered that

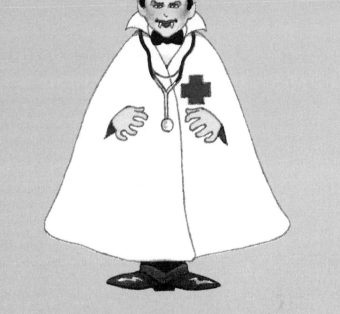

White Coat Hypertension

You can't always believe what a blood pressure gauge tells you. Sometimes the high numbers just indicate that you're nervous in the presence of a doctor. As a result, you may be diagnosed as hypertensive—and unnecessarily prescribed drugs—when your blood pressure is in fact much lower than it seems—or perfectly normal.

To avoid an error, your doctor should take 6 or 7 readings, 2 or 3 minutes apart, and average the last 3. And that procedure should be repeated on several visits before you're diagnosed as really having high blood pressure.

when potatoes are boiled, up to 50 percent of their potassium leaches out into the cooking water. Worse, the potatoes can absorb sodium that has been added to the pot. In contrast, steamed potatoes lost as little as 3 percent of their potassium and gained practically no sodium. The researchers say that steaming also conserves potassium in carrots, beans, peas, and fish, all rich sources of this mineral.

Next to potassium, calcium is probably the second most important mineral in blood pressure control. David A. McCarron, M.D., of the division of nephrology and hypertension at Oregon Health Sciences University in Portland, says that getting 1,000 milligrams of calcium a day can reduce the likelihood of developing high blood pressure from a 20 percent chance to a 1 percent chance. And taking calcium supplements is the easiest way to accomplish that, although most dairy products, greens and salmon can contribute enough calcium if a few servings are consumed daily.

Magnesium also helps to lower blood pressure, probably by interacting with potassium, sodium and calcium. When Swedish researchers gave magnesium supplements to 18 people being treated for high blood pressure, blood pressure fell significantly.

Another "soldier" in your dietary defense against high blood pressure is linoleic acid, found in vegetable oils such as sunflower and safflower oil but not in animal fats such as butter. Studies in the United States, Europe and India suggest that a diet rich in lino-

leic acid can lower blood pressure. One study showed that when people ate less dietary fat, with a larger proportion of what they *did* eat made up of polyunsaturated fat (high in linoleic acid) the subjects' blood pressure fell. When they resumed eating a diet high in fat but lower in polyunsaturated fat, their blood pressure rose.

Here are some other tips to lower high blood pressure.

Shed Those Pounds. It's common for blood pressure to rise when weight goes up and drop when pounds are shed. That may be because your sympathetic nervous system secretes increased adrenalinelike hormones as your weight goes up, resulting in elevated blood pressure. Another theory points the finger at additional fat cells, which decrease the effectiveness of insulin. To compensate, your body produces more insulin, resulting in increased sodium retention.

Anyone who has high blood pressure or a predisposition to it, and is also overweight, can do himself a big favor by slimming down.

Cork the Bottle. Drinking alcohol raises blood pressure by weakening the kidneys and stiffening the arteries. A survey of 83,947 people in the United States found that those who had three or more drinks a day had higher blood pressure than those who drank two or less drinks a day. The Framingham Heart Study—a major investigation of all facets of heart disease—revealed a similar link. And a British study found that of 132 alcoholics, over half had high blood pressure. In most patients, blood pressure fell when they stopped drinking, only to rise again when they returned to the bottle.

So if you have high blood pressure, cutting down (or cutting out) alcohol earns you one more notch in your belt in the fight against heart disease.

Snuff the Cigarette. Smoking is another accessory to the crime of high blood pressure. That is, while cigarettes may not directly cause high blood pressure, they contribute to the disease or make it worse.

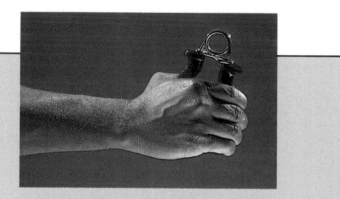

Tense Up to Relax

When you yawn and stretch, you're doing a kind of isometric exercise—tensing and relaxing your muscles.

Regular, daily isometrics (of a more structured kind) can lower your blood pressure, says Broino Kiveloff, M.D., of New York City. To perform isometrics:

1. Stand in a relaxed position.
2. Tense all your muscles as tightly as possible, without clenching your fists or bending your elbows. *Breathe normally* and count out loud, "One-one-thousand, two-one-thousand," to six-one-thousand.
3. Rest several seconds and repeat twice.
4. Do this 3 times a day.

Have Fun. Blood pressure control isn't all "don'ts." Some of the steps you can take are positive.

And the first step should be out the door and around the block a few times. The more you exercise, the less likely you are to gain weight. But exercise also seems to keep blood pressure low by making blood vessels more supple, elastic and resistant to the artery-hardening effects of age and arterial plaque buildup. Another theory suggests that exercise increases your body's ability to shift fluids out of circulation and into spaces between cells. When this happens, the volume of blood is decreased and your blood pressure is lowered. Studies have shown just how much exercise can help: After participating in an eight-week exercise program that included walking, cycling, jogging and other aerobic exercise, people studied at the Baylor College of Medicine in Houston had lower blood pressure than before. In another study, Harvard grads who exercised over the years had lower blood pressure than fellow alumni who didn't exercise, regardless of their age.

Handle Stress. Constant stress—or a panicky way of dealing with stress—may also aggravate high blood pressure. Evidently, suppressing anger or anxiety or other reactions to stress stirs up hormones called catecholamines. Scientists have a strong hunch that catecholamines raise blood pressure by tightening the blood vessel walls or by increasing the heart's output—or both.

The trick, then, is to find a way to take the edge off stress. Doctors often prescribe various methods of stress control—relaxation techniques, biofeedback and deep breathing, to name a few. These methods not only lower blood pressure for the time they're practiced, but also reduce tension—and blood pressure—around the clock.

You can choose the stress-coping technique that most appeals to you, because they all help to keep a lid on blood pressure.

Use Drugs as a Last Resort. All too often, the first thing a doctor does to correct high blood pressure is prescribe drugs—usually diuretics. These

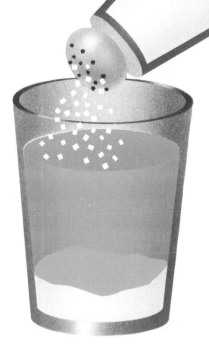

reduce blood pressure by flushing out water and sodium, thereby reducing the load on the heart and blood vessels. The trouble is, along with all that water and sodium a few other, critical minerals also get flushed away, mainly potassium, magnesium and calcium. Even more serious, diuretics can raise cholesterol levels, decrease glucose tolerance (hazardous if you are diabetic) and raise uric acid levels (predisposing you to gout.) Diuretics also are associated with digestive problems and can reduce both sexual drive and performance in men.

If diuretics don't bring down blood pressure, a doctor may prescribe beta-blockers. These slow down the heartbeat. Possible side effects are depression, drowsiness, hallucinations, cold hands and feet and allergic disorders. More seriously, they can aggravate congestive heart failure. And they raise blood levels of triglycerides and lower high-density lipoprotein (HDL) cholesterol, thereby *increasing* your chances of heart disease!

The next medical recourse is the use of arteriolar dilators—drugs that widen narrowed arteries and ease blood flow. Possible side effects include gastrointestinal disturbances,

Soft Water: How Much Salt Is Added?

Softening water by exchanging the hardness of minerals for sodium may create serious problems for those with high blood pressure. For example, treating water that is moderately hard (3 to 6 grains per gallon) can add as much as 40 milligrams of salt to each quart of water. If your water is very hard (12 to 30 grains per gallon) you may be adding as much as 225 milligrams of salt to each quart.

Therefore, hook the softener only to the hot water system and use cold water for drinking and cooking, or soften all the water in the house except the water to the kitchen sink.

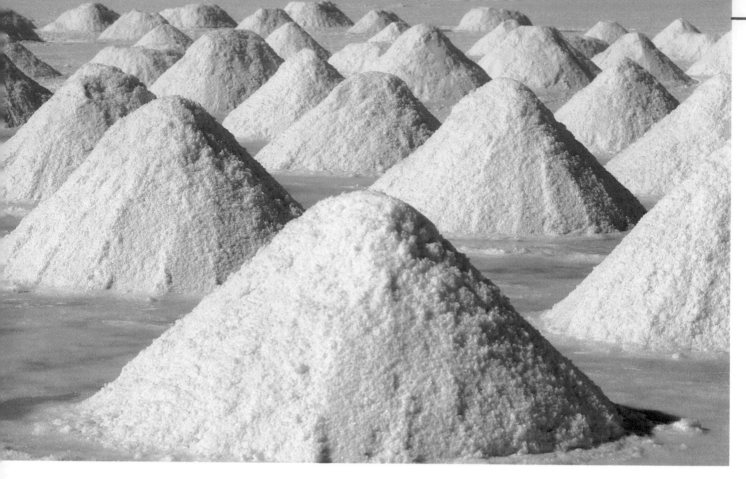

Salt has always been a staple of the world's diet. Mined by the ton—here from the salt lake Salar de Uyuni, Bolivia—it soon becomes only a sprinkle of white across the surface of a steak. Yet even that slight sprinkle can be trouble for the person with high blood pressure.

aggravation of angina, headaches, dizziness, fluid retention, nasal congestion, rashes, hepatitis and hair growth on the face and body. Peripheral dilators also are used. Side effects from this set include fatigue, sluggish heartbeat, reduced exercise tolerance, diarrhea and other digestive complaints.

No matter which drugs are prescribed, up to one-half of the people who are supposed to take them simply don't. No wonder! The side effects can be bothersome *and* serious.

Luckily, nondrug methods may help control blood pressure *and* prevent coronary heart disease, without dangerous side effects. In one study, doctors found that two-thirds of a group of people with mild hypertension were weaned off drugs by losing weight, eating less sodium, drinking less alcohol and exercising more. The beauty of this is that nondrug techniques double as disease *prevention* for people who are susceptible to high blood pressure but are still healthy. But remember: your physician should guide you, regardless of the therapy you may prefer.

ATHEROSCLEROSIS: A TIGHT SITUATION

At one time or another, you've probably been caught in a traffic jam caused by a disabled vehicle on the expressway. Traffic is reduced to one lane. Drivers impatiently inch ahead, but get nowhere—and get angry. To make matters worse, some wise guy decides to pull into the breakdown lane, preventing the tow truck from getting through to remove the disabled car. Before long, traffic is at a complete standstill.

Atherosclerosis is much like a traffic jam in your arteries. First, during childhood and adolescence, fatty streaks develop on artery walls. By age 25, arteries are partially blocked with plaque (a sludge of fats such as cholesterol and triglycerides). The buildup in some areas snowballs, until by age 50 you may have arteries only half as wide as they were at age 25—in effect, reduced to one lane. Blood has a hard time traveling to the heart.

If a clot (thrombus) forms, the artery may be completely blocked.

Sometimes, small standby vessels open up to detour blood to the heart. Should that emergency procedure fail, however, blood no longer can deliver life-sustaining oxygen to the heart. Parts of the heart muscle die. That's called a heart attack.

No one knows what causes artery sludge. Several things seem to encourage the buildup, though. One is an inherited tendency to manufacture a lot of cholesterol, which clings to artery walls. High blood pressure, the most important risk factor for heart disease, encourages that buildup. So does cigarette smoking. Other risk factors are overweight, lack of exercise and diabetes, the latter because blood sugar abnormalities seem to promote the production of cholesterol. Stress, too, seems to add to the buildup in the arteries.

Another way to think about atherosclerosis is to compare it to the buildup of scale in household plumbing. Just as a sluggish tap is often caused by years of accumulation of pipe scale, a heart attack is the climax of years of artery sludge buildup. To solve your water problem, a plumber can replace all the pipes. But if you do nothing to reduce the amount of minerals in your water supply, the pipes will eventually clog up again. The same thing applies to the sludge in your arteries. You can undergo a coronary artery bypass operation, in which a surgeon takes blood vessels, usually from your leg, to give your heart new arteries. But surgery is a lot more serious than plumbing repairs—and costs thousands of dollars. If you do nothing to reduce future buildup of artery sludge, your "new" coronary arteries, too, will become clogged. Besides, the same process that pumps sludge into your coronary arteries is also blocking the arteries to your brain and other organs. So a coronary bypass may be a stop-gap measure, but it's not a solution.

No matter what your age, it's not too late to fix your arterial plumbing. Doctors report that atherosclerosis definitely can regress. In some people it can be stopped in its tracks. What do these people do that puts the brakes on arterial disease—or even reverses it? The same things you can do.

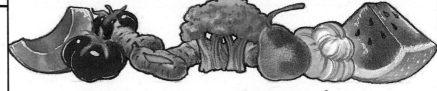

Food Sources of Potassium

Food	Portion	Potassium (mg.)
Potato	1 medium	782
Avocado	½ medium	602
Raisins	½ cup	545
Sardines, Atlantic, drained solids	3 oz.	501
Flounder	3 oz.	498
Orange juice	1 cup	496
Broccoli, raw	1 medium stalk	481
Squash, winter	½ cup	473
Banana	1 medium	451
Apricots, dried	¼ cup	448
Tomato, raw	1 medium	444
Watermelon	1 slice	426
Cantaloupe	¼ medium	413
Milk, skim	1 cup	406
Salmon, fillet, fresh, cooked	3 oz.	378
Great Northern beans, cooked	½ cup	374
Buttermilk	1 cup	371
Milk, whole	1 cup	370
Cod	3 oz.	345
Sweet potato	1 medium	342
Beef liver	3 oz.	323
Apricots, fresh	3 medium	313
Sirloin steak, trimmed of fat	3 oz.	307
Round steak, trimmed of fat	3 oz.	298
Haddock	3 oz.	297
Pork, trimmed of fat	3 oz.	283
Leg of lamb, trimmed of fat	3 oz.	274
Turkey	3 oz.	255
Perch	3 oz.	243
Tuna, drained solids	3 oz.	225
Chicken	3 oz.	196

Give Up Cigarettes. People with clean arteries don't smoke. Smoke is pure poison for coronary arteries. Researchers at the University of Southern California School of Medicine have found that nicotine-containing cigarettes stunt production of a substance called prostacyclin (PGI_2) in blood vessels, thereby accelerating artery disease. And when British researchers compared the arteries of 38 smokers with those of 14 nonsmokers who'd had coronary bypass operations, they found that the smokers' arteries were far more clogged than were the nonsmokers' arteries.

If you've had a heart attack or a coronary bypass, the first step to recovery is to throw your cigarettes in the trash. Switching to low-tar, low-nicotine brands won't do the trick, either. People who smoke so-called "safer" cigarettes still have up to a 75 percent higher death rate than nonsmokers. So the only truly safe cigarette is one that's not lit.

Change Your Diet. Since eating a lot of fat and cholesterol promotes heart disease, it's logical that eating less fat and cholesterol prevents heart disease. Better yet, a low-fat diet can *reverse* existing atherosclerosis. Studies with monkeys and other animals have proven that plaques induced by high-cholesterol diets shrink or disappear when the animals eat lower amounts of fat and cholesterol.

How do you cut the fat? It's much easier than you might think. Start by trimming away all visible fat from steaks, roasts and chops. (You can wait until after the meat is cooked, since fat does seal in moisture and flavor.) Buy the leanest ground beef you can find.

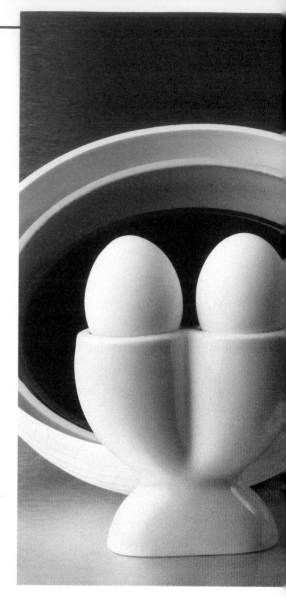

Atherosclerosis begins when the inner lining of artery walls is stripped away, leaving bare patches. Cells deeper within the wall then begin to multiply at those patches, forming niches that accumulate blood fats, particularly cholesterol. Those accumulations (called plaque) eventually thicken and block the flow of blood—usually by snagging blood clots that circulate through blood vessels. The walls of these diseased arteries also harden with deposits of calcium, which then raises blood pressure within them.

When blood flow is severely blocked by atherosclerosis, the tissues beyond the blockage die from lack of oxygen, causing a heart attack or a stroke.

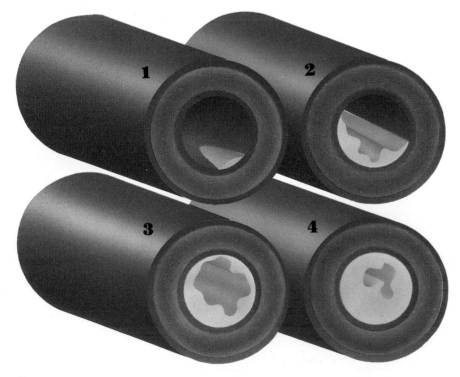

Eat less beef and pork and more veal, fish and fowl, which are lower in saturated fats. Remove the skin from chicken. Choose white meat over dark. Avoid sausage, frankfurters and cold cuts, which are high in fat.

When cooking meat, fish or fowl, boil, broil, bake, stew or braise—don't fry. And plan to go "meatless" one day a week.

Poach or boil eggs instead of scrambling or frying them to eliminate the need for cooking in fat.

Cut down on baked goods, which usually contain milk, eggs, butter and sugar, which has also been indirectly linked to heart disease. And scrutinize labels of nondairy creamers and other packaged foods for coconut oil, a highly saturated vegetable fat that clings to your arteries like glue.

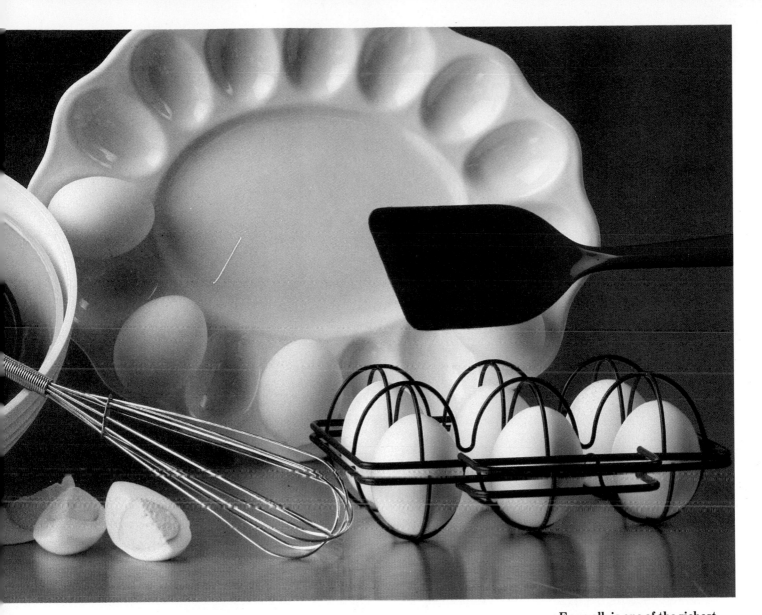

Be aware that not all dietary fats are bad for you. Different fractions of blood fat do different things to your arteries. Low-density lipoprotein (LDL) cholesterol mucks up arteries, while high-density lipoprotein (HDL) cholesterol keeps arteries free of plaque. In fact, fish and vegetable oils are good guys, so of the fat you do eat, most should come from these oils. For one thing, vegetable oils have no cholesterol and both types of oil are polyunsaturated, so they don't turn into artery sludge as readily as animal fats. Scientists have also discovered that fish and vegetable oils may actually be beneficial to the heart and arteries.

The heart-saver ingredients in fish oils are EPA oils, the primary one being eicosapentaenoic acid (also called EPA). Notably, salmon, mackerel, sardines, trout and haddock are highest in EPA oils.

Doctors first became interested in the protective effect of fish oils when they noticed that Eskimos and other people in fishing villages, who subsisted on large quantities of fish, rarely had heart disease. Further studies have since shown that by supplementing the diet with fish or fish oil, almost anyone can reap the same benefits.

Two British cardiologists gave supplements containing EPA to 150 people, many of whom had heart disease. After two years of supplementation, triglycerides and total cholesterol fell and HDL cholesterol (the good kind) rose—producing the same healthful condition found in Eskimos.

Fish is available in numerous varieties. And for convenience, you can also buy fish oil in capsules.

(continued on page 12)

Egg yolk is one of the richest sources of cholesterol. Some researchers have found that eating eggs raises blood cholesterol. Others say eggs have no effect. Should you eat them or not?

To be on the safe side, people with heart disease or a family history of it should probably steer clear of them. Otherwise, most research suggests it's safe to enjoy eggs in moderation— once or twice a week.

Foods That Keep the Ticker Ticking

Good heart health is a matter of adding the right foods to your diet, not just giving up sinful favorites. Salmon, poultry, broccoli, yogurt, citrus fruits, soybeans, kale and potatoes are chock full of one or more nutrients that help dissolve blood clots, lower cholesterol or control blood pressure. Cheeses that are high in calcium but also low in cholesterol help keep the lid on blood pressure. Onions and garlic keep blood thin and flowing, so it's less prone to clot. Melons are storehouses of vitamin C, which raises the levels of HDL (good cholesterol) and lowers LDL (bad cholesterol). Nuts, molasses, brown rice and soybeans all supply a hearty amount of magnesium, which also helps lower your blood pressure.

Cold Oriental Black Sea Bass

The fats found in fish can prevent blood platelets from sticking together, and thus help prevent heart attacks and strokes.

Serve this recipe with hot brown rice and lightly steamed snow peas.

Makes 4 to 5 servings

1 tablespoon peanut
    oil
3 cloves garlic
1 medium onion,
    thinly sliced
5 thin slices peeled
    ginger root
1 cup water

1½ cups rice wine
    vinegar
1 teaspoon turmeric
2½ pounds black sea
    bass fillets,
    skinned and cut
    into 1-inch strips
1 teaspoon tamari soy
    sauce

In a heavy skillet, heat oil and saute garlic, onion and ginger for 2 minutes, stirring constantly. Remove skillet from heat and add water, vinegar and turmeric.

Return to heat and bring liquid to a boil. Add fish to liquid. Lower heat to a very slow simmer. Cover and poach for 6 to 8 minutes. Cool in liquid and add tamari.

Refrigerate for 24 hours in liquid before serving.

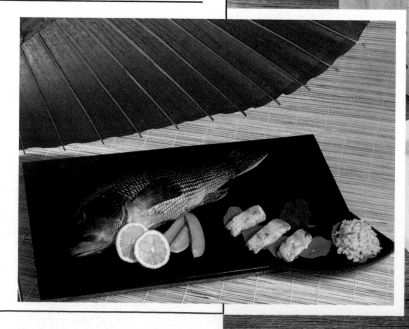

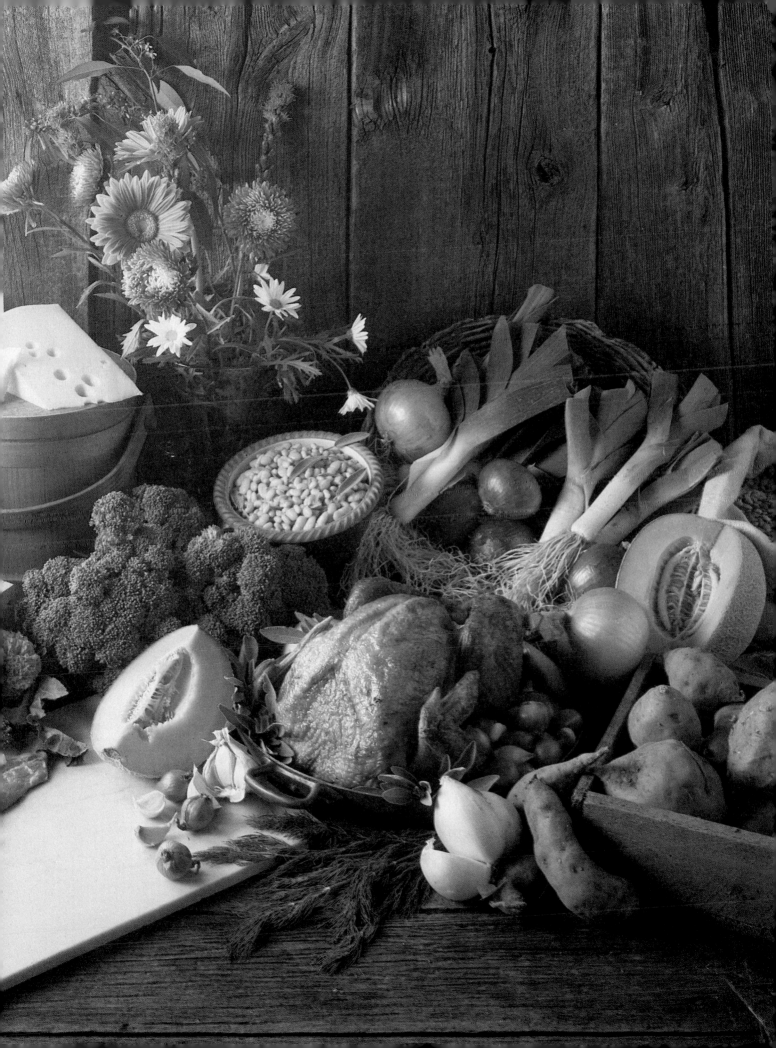

The secret weapons in vegetable oils are two essential fatty acids, linoleic acid and linolenic acid. Linoleic acid lowers blood pressure, and linolenic acid is believed to be converted to eicosapentaenoic acid in the body. The result? Less chance of a heart attack.

Polyunsaturated oils containing these fatty acids are generally found in vegetables, especially grains, nuts and seeds. (They also are found in fish.) Using sunflower, safflower, corn or soy oil for cooking and salad dressings will also supply generous amounts. In one study, a group of French farm families substituted oils and margarine containing linoleic and linolenic acids for butter. As a result, their blood had a far less pronounced tendency to clot, lowering their risk of heart disease.

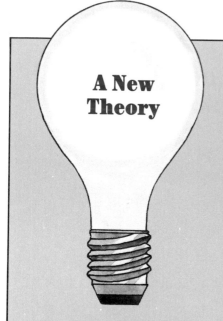

A New Theory

What actually causes artery sludge? Kilmer McCully, M.D., a pathology professor at Harvard Medical School, thinks that atherosclerosis is the end result of a series of events triggered by a deficiency of vitamin B6.

According to Dr. McCully, the original lesion, or plaque deposit, is caused by a toxic substance, homocysteine. When B6 is present, homocysteine is unable to do its destructive work. B6 defuses homocysteine by facilitating an enzyme action that converts homocysteine into cystathione, a safe, nontoxic substance.

Dr. McCully feels that because B6 is necessary to prevent the buildup of homocysteine in the blood, the vitamin can do much to prevent the original lesion leading to artery disease.

Beans, peas, nuts, grains, bananas and avocados are good sources of B6.

Consider Taking Supplements. For example, lecithin works wonders. A natural substance found in the oil of soybeans, lecithin lowers the concentrations of cholesterol and other fats in the blood. That was first discovered by Los Angeles physician Lester Morrison, M.D., D.Sc., who tried it on a group of people with high cholesterol who did not respond to a low-fat diet or other attempts to lower blood fats. Dr. Morrison added 2 tablespoons of lecithin, three times a day (a total of 36 grams per day) to their regimen. After three months, 12 out of 15 people had striking reductions in blood cholesterol. Later studies using comparable amounts of lecithin have supported Dr. Morrison's conclusions.

In addition to lecithin, certain vitamins and minerals seem to help arteries stay free and clear of sludge buildup. In large doses—quantities in which it cannot be used without a doctor's supervision—niacin reduces triglyceride production, lowers cholesterol and raises HDL cholesterol. However, because such high doses of niacin make blood vessels dilate and cause the skin to suddenly flush shortly after it's taken, most doctors don't prescribe it. If you decide to take niacin, don't do so on your own, but take the time to find a doctor who will cooperate with and supervise this treatment.

Also consider vitamin C (ascorbic acid). In one study of 150 people, blood tests showed that those people with atherosclerosis had far less vitamin C in their blood cells than people free of the disease. Because vitamin C plays a role in fat metabolism and other biological processes related to artery disease, cardiologists at the University of Louisville feel that vitamin C deficiency may play some role in the development of heart disease.

Other doctors are convinced that extra vitamin C can ward off heart disease—or stop it in its tracks—by lowering blood fats, by making blood platelets less "sticky" and by increasing fibrinolytic activity (the rate at which blood clots are dissolved). In one study, doctors gave 1,000 milligrams of vitamin C a day to 19 people with high cholesterol and 24 with high triglycerides.

Blood levels of both types of fats fell and blood levels of vitamin C increased. In another study, doctors gave 40 heart attack victims 2,000 milligrams of vitamin C a day, divided into two doses. Cholesterol dropped by 12 percent and platelet "stickiness" fell by 27 percent. In another phase of that same study, fibrinolytic activity rose by 62.5 percent. All those effects reduce the chances of formation of heart-threatening clot.

Low vitamin C levels may explain why smokers have more heart disease than nonsmokers: Smoking is known to lower blood levels of vitamin C.

Of all the minerals known to be essential to health, chromium is possibly the most promising as a plaque fighter. Howard A. I. Newman, Ph.D., a professor of pathology at Ohio State University College of Medicine, found that people with heart and artery disease have less chromium in their blood and blood vessels than people with healthy arteries.

Since too much sugar and other refined carbohydrates in the diet can flush chromium from the body, people concerned with mending their arteries should avoid sweets and highly processed baked goods and supplement their diet with brewer's yeast, the most reliable source of chromium.

Vitamin E lowers your chances of heart disease by raising HDL cholesterol. In a study by Robert London, M.D., head of the division of clinical research at Sinai Hospital in Baltimore, everyone who took the vitamin experienced a rise in HDL cholesterol in their blood. In another study, a group of Milwaukee researchers supplemented 43 people with 800 international units (I.U.) of vitamin E per day for four weeks. The people who had the lowest HDL levels improved the most.

Exercise for Your Heart's Content. Sitting on your duff all day contributes more to heart disease than you might think. And when inactivity is combined with other risk factors, some people might as well cement the sludge to their artery walls. Exercise, on the other hand, seems to break down plaque and flush it out.

Studies have shown that regular activity shuttles cholesterol to the liver, where it can be disposed of. And exercise can lower triglycerides, another type of blood fat that mucks up arteries. Even better, exercise raises blood levels of HDL cholesterol. Regular workouts, therefore, are especially beneficial for men and for women past menopause, who have less HDL cholesterol in their blood than premenopausal women. Exercise also helps to dissolve any blood clots—the "plugs" that often cause heart attacks.

Exercise can strengthen the heart muscle itself, conditioning it to pump more efficiently. It may also lower blood pressure, help to control weight and ease tension.

And here's a pleasant surprise: You don't have to go into Olympic training to achieve these wonderful health benefits. Researchers in Finland found that mild to moderate exercise (three or four times a week) lowered triglycerides and raised the protective HDL cholesterol in half the members of a group of middle-aged men. Blood fats in the other half of the group didn't change. Writing in the journal *Circulation*, the researchers commented that exercise is good not only for preventing coronary heart disease but also possibly for treating it.

How hard, *exactly*, must you exercise? The consensus is that three 20- to 30-minute sessions a week—whenever you can fit them into your schedule—are adequate.

And here's *another* nice surprise: You don't have to run or jog.

"Walking is as good as jogging," says Dan Streja, M.D., of the department of medicine at the University of Manitoba in Winnipeg, Canada. "To favorably alter cholesterol . . . and triglycerides and to lose weight, walking will do it."

Dr. Streja and another doctor did a study that showed that all sorts of good things happened to the blood chemistry of middle-aged men with heart disease who went on a walking program—and they only had to walk an average of three times a week for an average distance of just under 1¾ miles.

Whatever type of exercise you select, the cardinal rule for anyone is

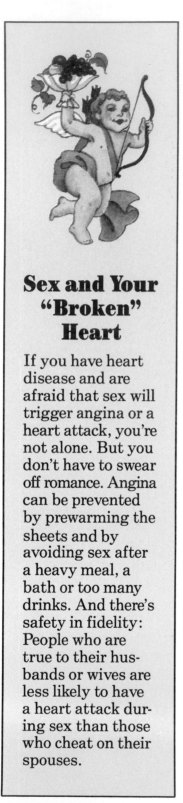

Sex and Your "Broken" Heart

If you have heart disease and are afraid that sex will trigger angina or a heart attack, you're not alone. But you don't have to swear off romance. Angina can be prevented by prewarming the sheets and by avoiding sex after a heavy meal, a bath or too many drinks. And there's safety in fidelity: People who are true to their husbands or wives are less likely to have a heart attack during sex than those who cheat on their spouses.

"Joiners" live longer than loners, according to a study of 6,928 residents of Alameda County, California. Keeping in close touch with friends and family does your heart good. Here 3 generations of lovely women share a close moment.

to start slow and take it easy. Warm up for 5 to 10 minutes first. Don't exercise when you're tired or when it's very hot or cold. And stop at once if you feel dizzy or have chest pains. After your workout, taper off for 10 minutes. Walk around. Abrupt halts trap too much blood in the lower body muscles, stymieing circulation to the heart.

ARE YOU THE CORONARY TYPE?

MAN: We Type A people really accomplish a lot.

WOMAN: We have to—we don't live as long as other people.

That brief exchange actually took place, and both people may be right. Several years ago, two astute San Francisco physicians, Ray H. Rosenman, M.D., and Meyer Friedman, M.D., noticed that people seem to be divided into two main behavior types: the hurried, driven, impatient, competitive Type A's and the unruffled, patient and more satisfied Type B's. The doctors also noticed that Type A people suffer two to three times more heart disease than Type B people. Since this discovery, a number of doctors have formally linked the two types of behavior to people who do and don't get heart attacks. Time-driven, success-conscious behavior could drive people to an early grave.

No one knows how this compulsive behavior fosters atherosclerosis, but doctors suspect it has something to do with how Type A people respond to stress. Presumably, they let stress overstimulate their nervous system, which in turn may promote buildup of artery sludge and trigger arterial spasms, two characteristic features of heart disease. Type A people also have a higher level of cholesterol in their blood—a major risk factor for heart disease.

Which are you, an A or a B? Do you usually:

- Find it difficult to sit still or relax, even when on vacation?

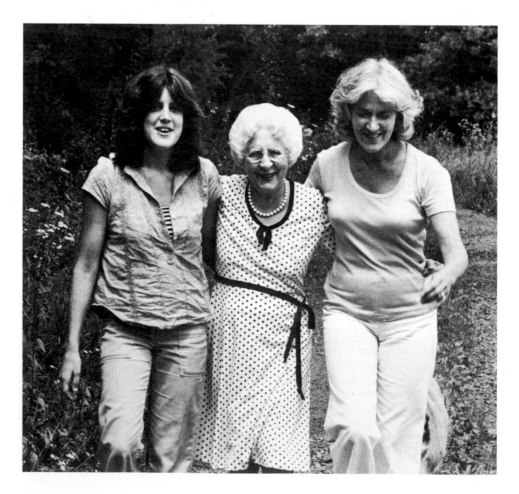

- Like to do several things at once?
- Drive, work, eat and speak faster than most other people?
- Repeatedly tap, drum or shake your hands or feet, or otherwise fidget?
- Interrupt others or finish their sentences for them?
- Often hear yourself described as a workaholic?
- Feel hostile or angry much of the time?

If you answer yes to most of those questions, you may very well be a Type A. If not, you're probably a Type B.

How can a leopard change its spots? Doctors feel that for anyone who's already had a heart attack, it's just as important to change stress-addicted behavior as it is to change your diet, to start exercising or to stop smoking. But you don't have to wait for a heart attack to scare you out of your Type A ways. Here's how to change this dangerous behavior *now.*

- Don't overreact.
- Set more realistic goals for yourself.
- Lower your expectations of others.
- Judge your life more on quality than by how much you produce.
- Look for humor in the things that make you angry.
- Take delays in stride.
- Try to cut down on or eliminate coffee, tea and cigarettes.
- Practice a relaxation technique.
- Exercise.

A STROKE: OXYGEN STARVATION FOR THE BRAIN

A stroke is an interruption of the blood supply to the brain. The most common type of stroke—cerebral thrombosis—occurs when a clot forms inside an artery that supplies blood to the brain. Another form—cerebral embolism—occurs when a clot wanders through the blood-stream and wedges itself in one of the arteries to the brain. A cerebral hemorrhage occurs when an artery ruptures and blood overflows into brain tissue.

Regardless of the type of stroke, the result is the same: brain damage due to oxygen and nutrient starvation. If enough of the brain is injured, a stroke can be fatal.

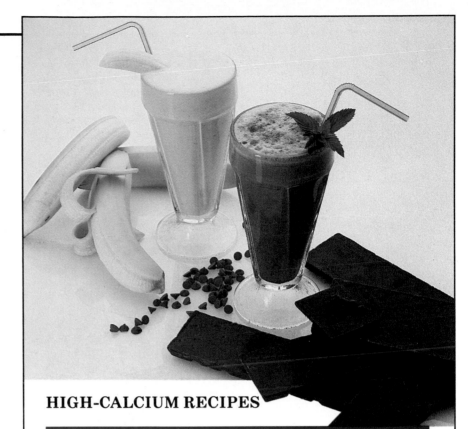

HIGH-CALCIUM RECIPES

Brown Velvet

Makes 2 servings

2 cups low fat milk
¼ cup carob powder
2 tablespoons nonfat dry milk
2 teaspoons brewer's yeast
½ teaspoon vanilla

Combine ingredients in blender container and whiz for 1 minute. Each serving provides 500 milligrams of calcium and 183 calories.

Banana Smoothie

Makes 2 servings

2 cups buttermilk
2 large bananas

Combine ingredients in blender container. Whiz until smooth and foamy. Each serving provides 292 milligrams of calcium and 204 calories.

15

Because most strokes are caused by high blood pressure and atherosclerosis, controlling these diseases also helps prevent strokes and possibly speed recovery. Exercise and other physical activity is especially helpful, because it improves fibrinolytic activity—the rate at which blood clots are dissolved. It's also vital that physical rehabilitation begin as soon as possible, to increase circulation and maintain flexibility. Then, when the brain has recovered, the muscles and joints will be ready, willing and able to comply with the directions they receive. While the brain is healing, the disabled muscles must be exercised or they will lock up and resist movement.

A fish-oil capsule a day keeps the clots away—by making blood platelets less "sticky." Garlic oil helps, too—by preventing clots from forming.

To break up the clots that caused a stroke, doctors give clot-dissolving medicines, called thrombolytic drugs, intravenously. Afterward, anticoagulants sometimes are prescribed to prevent further clots from forming. The drawback is that people taking these drugs bleed freely. Because of their side effects, anticoagulants are best used only during the first few months after a stroke, when the risk of clotting is highest. If you're taking fish oil or garlic oil, let your doctor know so that he can adjust your dosage of anticoagulant drugs, if necessary.

A stroke isn't always a bolt out of the blue. Very often, warning signals, or "mini-strokes," appear days, weeks or months before. If you experience a mini-stroke, or any of the following symptoms, call your doctor. Prompt attention to these symptoms, outlined in the American Heart Association's book *Heart Facts*, can save your life.

- "Sudden, temporary weakness or numbness of the face, arm and leg on one side of the body.
- Temporary loss of speech, or trouble speaking or understanding speech.
- Temporary dimness or loss of vision, particularly in one eye.
- Unexplained dizziness, unsteadiness or sudden falls."

THROMBOPHLEBITIS: CLOTS IN THE VEINS

If the deep veins of the leg flare up and develop a clot, you've got thrombophlebitis. And if that clot chokes off blood flow or travels to the heart, lungs or brain, you've got big trouble.

Clots are most apt to arise if you don't move your legs for long periods: for instance, after surgery and maybe even on a cross-continental airplane trip, or sitting at your job all day. Women who take oral contraceptives are somewhat more prone to clots than others because of changes in blood chemistry caused by the Pill.

If a clot lodges deep in your veins, you'll be given medication to prevent more clots from forming or keep the existing clot from growing.

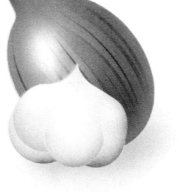

Take Two Onions . . .

People with phlebitis or other circulatory problems might benefit by learning to love the pungent flavor of garlic and onions.

Garlic oil contains 2 substances that prevent blood platelets from sticking together and forming clots. In one study, a doctor gave 25 milligrams daily of essential oil of garlic to 6 people. After 5 days, their blood was less quick to clot.

Both onions and garlic contain a substance that enhances fibrinolytic activity, the rate at which blood clots are dissolved.

Heavy use of garlic and onions in the Mediterranean area may explain why fewer people there die of heart attacks.

While the medication does its job, you will have to remain immobile to prevent the clot from traveling dangerously near vital organs.

To prevent clots, move around as much as possible. If you're confined to bed, "walk" against a pillow propped against the foot of the bed. If you're holed up in an airplane for hours, stretch and flex your legs and rotate your feet and lower legs as you sit. Do the same things at your work station, and take a stroll on your coffee breaks and at lunchtime.

Apart from those blood-pumping tactics, regular exercise helps to discourage clots by stimulating fibrinolytic activity. So does spicing your food with hot peppers, which contain substances that disperse clots.

ANGINA: A PAINFUL SYMPTOM

Angina is not a disease, but a symptom. When the heart has been deprived of oxygen for a few minutes—because of clogged arteries due to heart disease, an aorta narrowed by emotional upset or even because of anemia—the stabbing pain of angina occurs. This pain may feel different to different people. Sometimes the pain feels like indigestion, or it may start as an ache, perhaps in the arms.

Angina usually arises whenever the heart requires more oxygen than narrowed arteries can provide—for example, when you exert yourself, or when you feel cold. Angina is frightening, to be sure—but manageable. Here are a few tips to keep it under control.

Slenderize. Fewer pounds to tote around mean that your heart has less work to do and needs less oxygen. So if you lose weight, you'll have fewer angina episodes.

Quit smoking. Nicotine in cigarettes increases the heart's need for oxygen. At the same time, the carbon monoxide in cigarette smoke replaces oxygen molecules. The result: angina.

Breathe deeply. A Minnesota doctor found that slow, deep diaphragmatic breathing can ward off an angina attack. Fill your lungs very gradually, until your chest is fully expanded. Pause briefly. Then completely empty your lungs very, very slowly.

Exercise. We don't mean run the 50-yard dash. But a well-planned, regular exercise program slows the heart rate and decreases its oxygen requirements, making the heart more efficient and less prone to angina.

To avoid angina triggered by exertion, any physical activity must begin with fairly light exercise and progress slowly to more demanding tasks.

Ease up on alcohol. A couple of drinks may make you an easy mark for angina. In one study, alcohol increased the heart's demand for oxygen by speeding the heart rate and raising blood pressure. So if you have a couple of beers and then decide to play Frisbee with your kids or trot out on the dance floor with your spouse, chances are angina will sneak up on you more readily than if you engage in those efforts with no alcohol under your belt.

Eat more fish. Fish-oil supplements containing EPA increased exercise tolerance and reduced the need for nitroglycerin (a drug routinely prescribed for angina) in 150 people studied by British cardiologists.

By following a carefully worked plan to alter your diet, your exercise patterns and your lifestyle, angina pain may become just a bad memory.

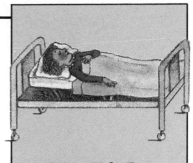

The Right Slant on Sleep

Angina may strike while you sleep—presumably because lying flat increases the amount of blood returning to the heart. Tilting the head of the bed up at a 10-degree angle reduces this flow and eliminates both the angina and the need for anti-angina drugs. Israeli doctors successfully used the technique to treat 8 people bothered by nighttime angina attacks.

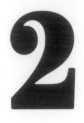

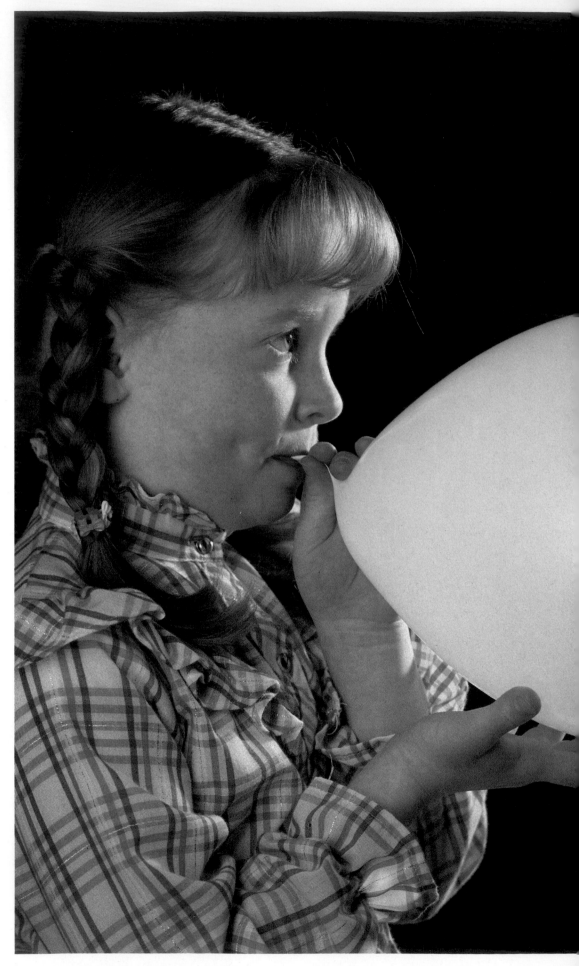

Help for Troubled Breathing

Smart choices in lifestyle are your surest defense against breathing disorders.

To blow on a dandelion puff and send your wishes flying across open space: What a pleasure! Yet open space can be loaded with pollen, and breathing can sometimes be a real struggle. But you can win that battle by adopting a game plan that is patterned on the process of breathing itself.

"In comes the good air; out goes the bad air." You can make that automatic reflex the basis for *choice*. Learn to take into your life what helps, and reject what hurts. Your initial choices are especially important. If you make choices that produce results, you'll find them much easier to repeat in the future—and it will be easy to build on your success.

These choices can have a positive impact on a wide variety of breathing-related disorders.

Your asthma attacks, for instance, could be triggered by something as simple as an unsuspected food allergy. Saying no to eggs for breakfast could end your problem. Do you suffer from emphysema? Understandably, you may be reluctant to exercise—after all, who wants to be *more* breathless? But once you say yes to exertion, the difference in your health may be dramatic.

Who wouldn't experiment with a change in diet if they knew it could ease congestion? And how many people would bother getting injected with pneumonia vaccine if they knew that they could get much better, and perhaps safer, protection simply by eating foods that strengthen the immune system?

Well-informed choices in your lifestyle can strengthen your body's natural healing powers. In many cases they can, of course, prevent problems from developing. Fortunately, they also can help to minimize a disease that's already "in progress." Now is the time to begin designing the custom-made program your body needs to breathe easier. And if, when you blew on that dandelion, your wish was for good health, it now may come true.

19

FINDING THE CAUSE OF ASTHMA

One of the scariest things about asthma is that you never know whether an attack will bring on only mild wheezing or develop into a serious emergency. Statistics show that asthma is seldom fatal. But when you're the one under attack, it can *feel* like you're dying—drowning in deep water. And just as though you were drowning, the more you panic the greater the danger.

What causes these terrifying attacks? In a general sense, the cause is the same for every one of the nine million Americans who suffer from asthma: Extra-sensitive muscles in

the bronchial tubes that tend to twitch. As they go into full-fledged spasm, air passages often clog up with mucus. Then the gasping begins.

Many doctors treat asthma by using drugs to stop the bronchospasm, and thus the wheezing. But a more effective approach is to prevent attacks in the first place. There's always something specific that triggers sensitive lungs into spasm. "Don't give up on finding those triggers," advises one doctor. "Where there's wheezing, there is always a cause."

Your attacks could start with pollen or mold spores, or with any of the environmental allergens that set off hay fever. (The difference between asthma and hay fever is that the

Pollen Concentrations in the United States

If pollen makes you wheeze, the circles on this map mean trouble. Yellow circles mark the places where ragweed pollen is at its lowest concentration. Red areas represent bigger trouble—pollen concentrations up to 400 percent higher. The green circles, however, stand for the densest patches of all. If you live in locations marked in green you may have severe problems and find it necessary to take special precautions during pollen season—late summer and early fall.

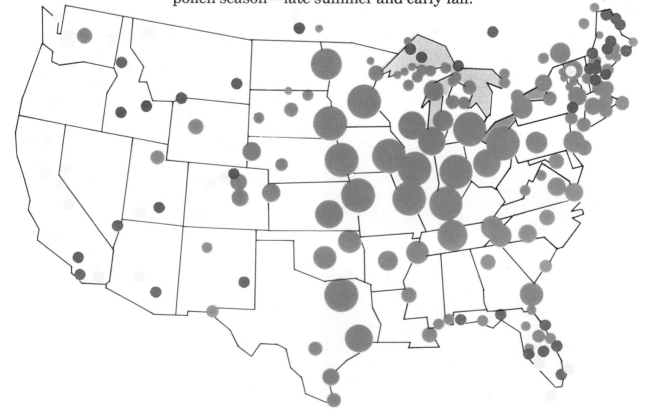

allergic reaction of asthma affects the lungs instead of the nose and eyes. However, hay fever sufferers may develop asthma later in life). Allergic reactions to food can also cause attacks. So can any kind of overstimulation: a strong odor, cold air, emotional upset, too much exercise. Even worse, two or more causes can team up to make an attack extra severe.

Thus, asthma isn't only a frightening disease; it can be terribly complicated. But if you are willing to persist until you dismantle every trigger for your attacks, you may be able to cure the disease permanently. Asthma can be completely reversible. And even if that's not possible in your case, natural remedies still may help you decrease your dependence on asthma medication.

THE HIDDEN TRIGGERS

Every night Bob had nightmares that he couldn't breathe. When he woke up, the nightmare didn't end. Asthma often forced Bob to leave his warm bed for the hospital emergency room. But despite the severity of his problem, Bob's attacks stopped completely once the cause was found: potatoes. Just one hidden food allergy started all those nightly attacks.

Breathing affected by eating? It's common, according to Bob's physician, James A. O'Shea, M.D., of Lawrence, Massachusetts. "Food allergies can be more complicated than, say, getting hives from eating strawberries," he says.

For some people, allergic reactions to food are a major cause of asthma. For others, food allergies combine with environmental allergies to make attacks more severe. For instance, dust may make you choke, but only when you have eaten eggs, thus weakening your system. And it may be easier to avoid eggs than to wipe the last speck of dust off the face of the earth.

If you'd like to see whether eliminating certain foods can help solve your asthma problem, you can get help from a specialist like Dr. O'Shea. (His specialty is called clinical ecology.) Or maybe you'd like

What Triggers Restaurant Asthma?

One minute Joan was savoring the restaurant's crisp salad. The next minute she couldn't breathe. What poisoned her into an asthma attack? A common preservative, metabisulfite, that keeps food looking garden fresh when it's long since out of the garden. Joan paid a pretty high price to have lettuce that didn't turn brown at the edges.

The kind of reaction Joan had is so common, doctors have named it "restaurant asthma." To keep that syndrome from ever becoming common in your life, it helps to know which restaurant foods are apt to have the highest concentrations: avocado dip, potatoes, salads, vegetables and shellfish. Unfortunately, the preservative isn't only in restaurant items. Wine and beer can contain metabisulfite. And at present, the U.S. Food and Drug Administration (FDA) allows its use, usually without labeling.

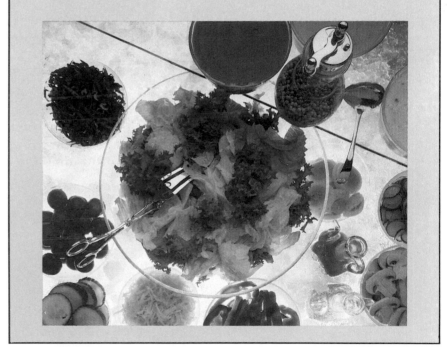

to do the detective work yourself. The first foods to investigate, according to Dr. O'Shea, are milk, corn, wheat, eggs, chocolate, citrus, beef, chicken and potatoes. But don't stop with these foods. Until your symptoms are gone completely, keep testing everything you eat or drink. Here's how to do it:

- Start keeping a log of your diet and health. Record every item you eat or drink and the time you do it. Also list any asthma episodes. All that notekeeping takes time, but it can reveal some patterns you'd otherwise miss. (In Bob's case, potatoes brought on asthma every time—but not until 7 hours after he ate them!)

- Eliminate one food from your diet completely for three weeks. If you don't cook every meal from scratch, read labels carefully. Pass up by-products of that food; for instance, cornstarch and corn syrup both count as corn.

- Resume eating the food with a generous serving at every meal for three days in a row. Two days later, analyze the results. If your asthma worsens after going back to a food, then that food is most likely an allergen. Remove it from your diet.

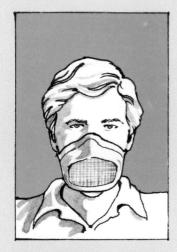

Air Filters for Easy Breathing

A simple surgical mask can screen out particles of dust, pollen and smoke. The mask also keeps *in* some of the air you've just breathed. This warm, moist air is so much easier to breathe, it can completely prevent wheezing—especially during exercise. In winter, you can get similar relief from chilly air by pulling a scarf over your nose and mouth.

All year around, your best protection indoors will come from a *good-quality* air filter. Quality matters, since some machines can be worse than useless. One specific filter is well worth its price, if you can afford it. HEPA (High-Efficiency Particulate Air) filters really do a heck of a job against airborne outsiders: 99.97 percent get zapped right out of action. Plug in a HEPA filter and, in a half hour or less, your asthma symptoms could be gone with the wind.

BREATHING AND NUTRITION

The next step you can take involves addition, not elimination. Medical researchers have found that vitamins B$_6$ (pyridoxine), C, A and D, and the mineral magnesium can all come to your aid.

During a five-month study reported in the *Annals of Allergy*, 38 children with moderate to severe asthma were given two 100-milligram supplements of B$_6$ daily. An equal number of other asthmatic youngsters received a placebo (a fake pill). Neither the doctors nor the kids were told who was getting which, but ongoing records were kept.

When the results were analyzed, it became clear that the vitamin takers had far fewer asthma attacks. Their breathing came easier and they needed less medication. Though this study measured results in children aged 2 to 16, it seems logical that adults would benefit, too. Keep in mind, however, that it took a full month for the benefits to materialize. (And also remember that the levels of B$_6$ used in this study should be taken only under a doctor's supervision.)

Another asthma stopper is vitamin C. In one study patients took 1 gram of vitamin C daily. As in the study with B$_6$, another group of people got a placebo. For the 14 weeks of the experiment, all asthma symptoms were recorded. The placebo group suffered 24 moderate to severe attacks. The group taking vitamin C had only 3. And when they stopped taking their supplements, their asthma came back within 8 weeks.

Dramatically freer breathing has also been gained by boosting intake of calcium plus vitamins D and A, according to research by Carl J. Reich, M.D., as reported in the *Journal of the International Academy of Preventive Medicine*. Among 10,000 patients treated, nutritional supplements reduced the severity of attacks—and even stopped some altogether—in 94 percent of asthma patients under 20 years of age, and in 77 percent of older people.

Dr. Reich says the treatment works because calcium improves lung functioning, vitamin D helps the body make use of that calcium and vitamin A keeps mucous membranes from overproducing.

Another nutritional defense against asthma may be too late to solve your problem but could help your *children.* Breastfeeding can counter the tendency for asthma to be hereditary. A study of babies of parents with allergies was reported in the *Lancet.* It found that those who were breastfed for their first six months showed a lower rate of allergy problems (including asthma) than formula-fed children.

ALLERGIC TO EXERCISE

People who suffer from the asthma triggered by overexertion are often understandably reluctant to exercise at all. But you don't have to avoid exercise, as long as you exercise some precautions along with your workout.

- Take vitamin C. Scientists at Yale found that 500-milligram doses, taken before workouts, reduce bronchospasm measurably.
- Warm up properly, so that your body can ease into a higher level of exertion.
- Breathe through your nose during and after exercise. When you keep your mouth closed, you switch on a kind of natural air-filtration system.
- Cool down your lungs after your workout with 5 to 10 minutes of diaphragmatic and pursed-lips breathing (see page 30).
- Select appropriate exercise. Sustained exertion most often causes spasms. Choose sports with built-in breathers, such as baseball. For noncompetitive exercise, try swimming. The warm temperature and moist air make breathing easier. (Avoid highly chlorinated pools, though; they can trigger an attack.)

LEARN TO RELAX

Because tension can contribute to the severity of an asthma attack, it's important to learn to relax. And

---

Relax Away Asthma

The American Lung Association teaches kids the following method to relax away asthma. It works well for adults, too. Practice for 5 minutes a day to train yourself to turn your body into a "wet noodle" at will. Once you're familiar enough with the feeling, it becomes easy to recognize and execute under other circumstances. Whenever you feel warning signs of an asthma attack coming on (such as a tight chest or shortness of breath), you will be able to relax your body in the same way. It can soothe an attack or prevent one completely.

1. Stand up straight. Make all your muscles very tight. Then take a deep breath. Point your chin to the ceiling and grit your teeth. Straighten your arms, lock your elbows and clench your fists. Stiffen your legs and toes. Pull in your stomach. Squeeze every muscle as stiff as you possibly can for about 3 seconds. Hold tight.

2. Release. Relax your muscles until you feel like a wet noodle, a rag doll—whatever is your favorite image of the ultimate in limpness. Enjoy the sensation.

3. Flop to the floor, stretch out and close your eyes. Keep everything limp and loose. Luxurious looseness. Feel it everywhere. Feet. Legs. Torso. Arms. Face.

4. Picture yourself floating down a river. Concentrate on your muscles one at a time. How delightfully relaxed they feel.

5. Breathe softly, easily, as though you were fast asleep in a cozy bed. Stay quiet for a while. Enjoy the pleasant sensation. That's the wet noodle feeling you want to remember.

---

there are numerous methods available to help you relax almost at will.

Biofeedback is one of those methods. It uses equipment to monitor how successful you are at relaxing. Feedback from the equipment, such as clicking noises, shows you which behavior to repeat. This method worked in a study of children with asthma, as reported in the *Annals of Allergy.* When the kids succeeded in relaxing their muscles, they were able to breathe more easily. To pursue this method, you'll need to purchase a biofeedback machine or locate a clinic that has one, and then take some special training.

Self-hypnosis is another do-it-yourself method that requires just a little expert training. One experiment, described in the *Journal of Allergy and Clinical Immunology,* showed that six teenagers with asthma were able to reduce the severity of their attacks after two months. By the next month, using self-hypnosis, they were also able to decrease the number of attacks.

Transcendental Meditation (TM) is another self-help for relaxation. This form of meditation is easy to master with less than a week of instruction.

CUSTOM-MAKE YOUR ENVIRONMENT

To cure asthma, patients in Poland have flocked to salt mines—and gotten good results. But you don't have to live in a mineshaft to escape your allergies. Try the following ways to make your situation more livable.

- Ask smokers to step outside.
- Exchange furry or feathered pets for an aquarium.
- To avoid stirring up mold, don't rake leaves or mow the lawn.
- Avoid products that contain

formaldehyde. These include foam insulation, laminated particle board, plywood and many rug and upholstery fabrics made of synthetic fibers.

- Refrain from eating foods that may contain FD&C Yellow No. 5 (tartrazine), including chewing gum, prepared macaroni and cheese and canned fruit and vegetables. Many other commercial products, from mouthwash to prescription drugs, also contain the dye.

- Drink up to a cup of liquid every hour to keep your airways moist. Hot beverages are the most soothing.

- Allergic reaction to aspirin is now known to cause as many as 20 percent of all asthma attacks. If you suspect your attacks may be linked to this painkiller, stop taking it. (What a cure! That's the kind of instant relief people expect to get from *taking* a pill.) Those who must use something like aspirin may be able to substitute an acetaminophen product like Tylenol.

- Avoid eyedrops with the ingredient timolol.

- Your asthma medicines also can represent danger. The problem with some of these medicines is that, though they relieve symptoms, they may bring along a host of side effects. For instance, long-term steroid use can cause cataracts and promote bone loss. Nor are problems limited to prescription drugs. Over-the-counter bronchodilators have the long-term effect of irritating the very tissues they are meant to clear. They may actually increase the number of attacks.

In an emergency, of course, asthma medication could save your life. And if a severe condition has been stabilized with drugs, it isn't prudent suddenly to throw them away. But given the danger of side effects, it's imperative that asthma drugs be used properly—in the smallest dose possible, for the shortest time possible and only when

Doctors are starting to get wind of the benefits of music. Children prefer practicing a woodwind or brass instrument instead of doing ordinary breathing exercises, yet it serves the same purpose: It relaxes breathing muscles.

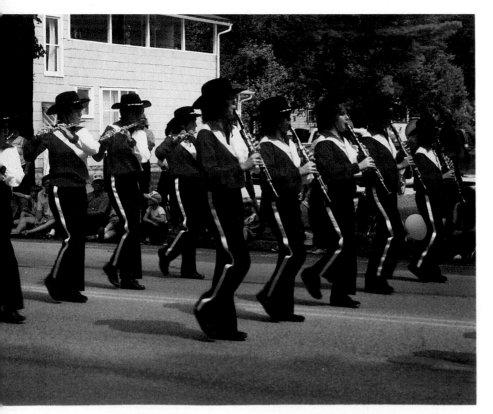

"Hay Fever"— All Four Seasons

Some allergens shift with the seasons. For example, spring's most likely troublemakers include tree and grass pollens. In summer, they're grass and weed pollens, along with mold and mildew. Fall's big culprit is the mold that comes from fallen leaves.

Although you'd think that winter is the safest season, it's not. The family pet and you spend more time indoors together, the furnace ducts are circulating dust and you're likely to get fumes from your furnace or kerosene heater.

nothing else works. Keep drugs at the minimum level by maximizing your nutrition, exercising with care and avoiding allergens.

PNEUMONIA—OLD AND NEW

America's number five killer could hardly be called a new disease—archaeologists have found the mummified remains of people who died of it 3,000 years ago. A lung infection, pneumonia usually starts with a virus or bacteria—but may even be caused by fungi (such as molds) and chemical irritants. Difficult breathing is one of the first symptoms, along with a dry cough and a fever.

But not all forms of pneumonia are this clear-cut. One type, which typically strikes young adults, is dangerous just because its victims don't realize they have it. "Walking pneumonia" masquerades as the flu. Without proper treatment, the immune system frequently remains weak, allowing for relapses that can be serious. So if in addition to a cough and a fever, you develop shortness of breath, check with a doctor to see if you have walking pneumonia.

A third form of the disease, considered new, made nationwide headlines in 1976 when 29 people staying at a plush hotel inexplicably died. Since most of the victims were attending an American Legion

convention, reporters dubbed their killer "Legionnaire's disease."

Medical detectives searched for six months before they tracked down the culprit: It was an unnamed organism that had been identified as early as 1947. Once its connection with Legionnaire's disease was known, it was named *Legionella pneumophila.* One of the sneakiest bacteria ever, it used to exist harmlessly in muddy outdoor places like streams. Then in 1976, it developed a new ability: It was able to move indoors. It found a new breeding ground in the unsanitary water in shower drains and air conditioners. And from these common household areas, it moves into its most preferred place of all—the human cells called macrophages. (Ironically, the whole purpose of macrophages is to defend the body against bacteria like *Legionella.*) This bug is most dangerous to people in poor health, and it finds 70,000 of them a year. It was no coincidence that the 29 people who died had in common smoking, drinking and generally weak immune systems; 4,400 other people attending the convention—as well as uncounted other visitors to the hotel—all were exposed to the same germs but left the hotel unscathed.

A weak immune system can set you up for all three kinds of pneumonia, but a strong one protects you. So keep that germ-fighting

Immunity for Your Lungs

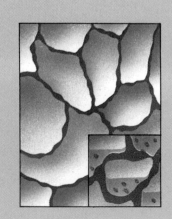

Alveoli, air sacs in the lungs, cluster like miniature grapes at the finest air passageways. When healthy, these "grapes" swell with oxygen, which gets passed along through capillaries and blood to the body's energy-hungry cells. In pneumonia (inset), bacteria or viruses clog up the alveoli with fluid.

There's a link between infected alveoli and a strained immune system, because the lungs are always open to attack from germs and toxins in the air we breathe. An overworked immune system doesn't defend as well, leaving the alveoli vulnerable to disease.

What puts a strain on immunity? Smoking. Drinking. Trying to recuperate from another illness. To fight off potential pneumonia, then, it pays to keep your resistance strong.

system strong by giving it the good nutrition it deserves.

ANTIOXIDANTS AND OTHER RESISTANCE BUILDERS

Antioxidants can be defined as "fighters of oxygen." But why should our immune systems need to fight this life-sustaining element? The oxygen we breathe reacts with chemicals inside the body to give us energy. But oxygen also reacts with other things in the body—specifically the fats found in cell membranes. This reaction can weaken and destroy the cell. And when those cells are the immune system's troubleshooting lymphocytes, your natural defenses also are weakened.

J. Terrel Hoffeld, D.D.S., Ph.D., with the National Institute of Dental Research, has specialized in studying the role antioxidants play in immunity. In the journal *Federation Proceedings,* he comments on his work:

"A whole series of biochemical reactions is involved [in oxidation]. If you can block those reactions in the early steps, then you can block the final result more efficiently. The most effective agent we found was vitamin E. It acts everywhere along the chain of steps, and therefore is very effective."

Some experts suggest that one daily 800-I.U. dose of vitamin E will keep you amply supplied. And while you're at it, they also suggest you supply yourself with another antioxidant, vitamin A. This nutrient magnifies vitamin E's effectiveness. In addition, vitamin A fights infection by building up some feisty members of the immune system, called lysozymes. Normally these are plentiful in the mucous membranes of your lungs, guarding them against invading viruses or bacteria that try to sneak in with the air you breathe. But without sufficient vitamin A, the lungs lose their lysozyme-rich mucus and fall prey to invaders.

Vitamin A can protect you from other assaults on the immune system as well. Both anesthesia and surgery depress your resistance and set you up for pneumonia. Steroid drugs also have the side effect of reducing immunity. And the sheer stress of living can rob you of up to 60 percent of your vitamin A, once again leaving you vulnerable. But you can avoid all these dangers with adequate vitamin A.

As with most good things, of course, too much of this vitamin can cause problems, because excess amounts of it get stored in the liver rather than flushed from the body. You won't have to worry about that, however, if you just follow some simple guidelines.

If you take your vitamin A in supplement form, don't exceed 25,000 I.U. per day without consulting your doctor.

Even better is to get your vitamin A straight from the food you eat. Good sources include liver, sweet potatoes, carrots, spinach, cantaloupe, kale, broccoli, winter squash and mustard greens. You're not likely to eat so many carrots you'd overdose on vitamin A— but you could eat enough to turn your skin orange.

What other nutrients can help you combat pneumonia by boosting resistance? Three B vitamins, perhaps: B_6, folate and pantothenate. Research published in the *Journal of the American Medical Association* showed that they are essential for the immune system's production of antibodies, those custom-made antidotes to different germs. Vitamin deficiencies slow down antibody production, but good nutrition can quickly bring it back to normal. You can get plenty of all the B vitamins by eating liver or brewer's yeast.

Besides fending off infection through antibodies and lysozymes, your immune system has another potent weapon: T-lymphocytes. These white blood cells destroy viruses— when they're functioning properly. For that, they need both vitamin C and zinc.

Your immune system is your best defense against pneumonia. Keep it nourished and healthy.

EASING BRONCHITIS AND EMPHYSEMA

It's a janitor's nightmare. Somehow the brooms have lost their power to clean. The bristles are too gummed up to sweep. Mopping works no better. The old dependable detergent doesn't clean any more. Even as you

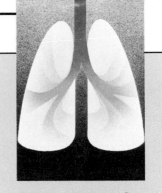

Pneumonia Vaccine?

Don't depend on vaccine to protect you from pneumonia. A review published by the *Journal of the American Medical Association* evaluated the evidence and concluded that pneumonia vaccines don't work, except for people with sickle cell anemia. For others, the one predictable result of vaccination is a 35 to 40 percent chance of side effects.

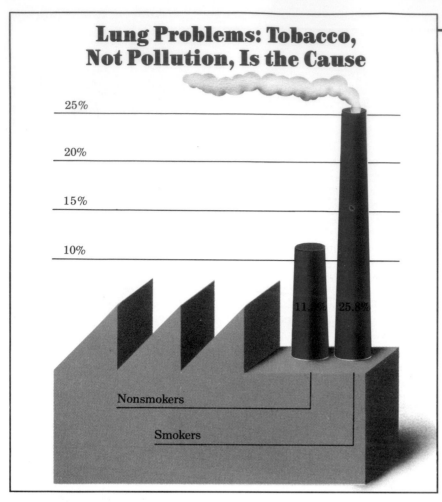

Lung Problems: Tobacco, Not Pollution, Is the Cause

25%

20%

15%

10%

11.2% 25.8%

Nonsmokers

Smokers

In a study done at an industrial medical center in France, researchers found that among the nearly 900 people tested for breathing capacity, the incidence of chronic respiratory problems among smokers was more than twice that among nonsmokers.

Researchers considered other factors, such as occupational exposure, housing, age and social class, and concluded that smoking—and no other factor—determined the frequency of symptoms.

scrub, the corroded linoleum grows stickier. Helplessness gradually gives way to sheer terror.

Such nightmares are a waking reality for those suffering from advanced Chronic Obstructive Lung Disease (C.O.L.D.)—the name used today by specialists when they speak of emphysema and chronic bronchitis.

With C.O.L.D., the "floor"—the lining of the lungs' air sacs—won't come clean. In cases of bronchitis, mucus production goes out of whack—there's too much of it, and it's the wrong consistency to perform its usual function of cleansing the airways. In fact, mucus itself may seem to be the enemy. It gets infected and thick, making you choke.

But you can ease congestion without resorting to drugs. Maintaining good nutrition, avoiding air pollution—especially smoke-filled rooms—and drinking plenty of water can add up to dramatic improvement in how you feel.

But the single biggest way you can help yourself is to stop smoking. It's almost always the cause of C.O.L.D. and the main factor that

aggravates the condition. There's no question that the best remedy for helping yourself is to quit.

While you're doing your best to break the addiction, however, there is something simple you can do to at least reduce the damage from tobacco smoke: Put down your cigarette between puffs. Research on 5,438 smokers, published in the *British Medical Journal,* showed that when you let a cigarette dangle from your lips instead of putting it down between puffs, you are much more likely to develop bronchitis.

And once you do manage to kick the habit, you'll soon notice that you cough less and breathe more freely. This improvement can be further accelerated with proper nutrition.

HOW TO STARVE A C.O.L.D.

With C.O.L.D., your respiratory and immune systems work overtime, making you extra vulnerable to other respiratory diseases. But you can protect yourself against these infections with proper nutrition.

If you could see what happens deep inside your body, you might compare infection to underwater survival, where big fish eat small ones. In your bloodstream, the defender cells of your immune system do battle with invading bacteria and viruses. What you eat can strengthen your defender cells so they become the "big fish," devouring predatory viruses and bacteria. And the "fish food" to use has these ingredients: zinc and vitamins A, C and E.

Zinc is vital for immunity because it nourishes lymphocyte cells that fight infection and helps the body to produce more antibody cells. You'll find zinc in wheat bran, wheat germ, green peas, lentils and popcorn.

Your menu also should include plenty of vitamin C. Even if you've quit, the smoking you did in the past may have created a deficiency of this important vitamin. It gets used up defending you against air pollution. Whether you smoke now or not, your lungs need its protection to fight respiratory infection. Also of primary importance to those with chronic breathing difficulties, particularly asthma, vitamin C acts as a natural antihistamine, reducing the swelling in your nasal passages and sinuses.

You can get plenty of vitamin C from citrus fruits, but don't neglect other excellent sources like red and green peppers, broccoli, brussels sprouts and kale. Ironically, the canned citrus juices you drink to stock up on vitamin C could be robbing your body of zinc; tin from the cans leaches into acidic juices and goes on to block zinc absorption. So if you want to drink your vitamin C, switch to fresh or frozen juices in cardboard containers.

Vitamin A fights many of the same bad guys as vitamin C. It can counter the effects of smoking and other pollutants, boost your overall immunity and even protect your lungs. You'll want to benefit from the way vitamin A teams up with zinc; zinc makes this vitamin perform more effectively. The best-known sources of vitamin A are the vivid green and orange vegetables. But don't slight lesser-known but excellent sources like peaches, apricots, red peppers and even cod-liver oil.

Add vitamin E for even more lung protection. This vitamin helps the lungs manufacture more defender cells. You'll get vitamin E into your diet with wheat germ, sunflower or corn oil, almost any type of nut, spinach, tomatoes, sweet potatoes and watercress.

Should you choose to use food supplements, the maximum amounts to take on your own are 500 milligrams of vitamin C, 30 milligrams of zinc, 25,000 I.U. of vitamin A and 800 I.U. of vitamin E. Levels higher than this should have your doctor's okay.

Saying yes to these nutrients can keep your respiratory problem under control, but you also need to learn to say no to a few things. When people around you have colds and flu, you've got to keep away—even if the sneezer is your best friend at work or your affectionate three-year-old.

HOUSEKEEPING HINTS FOR HEALTH

A good first step to make your home a healthier place is to rid it of breathing irritants. Start by cleaning your home heating system. Grimy equipment guarantees that you'll get dust to breathe along with the warmth. Besides contributing to your health problems, this dirt cuts heating efficiency, so cleaning up the mess can actually save you money. Therefore, once a year, hire a plumber or a heating service to clean the whole unit. At the same time, if your house is heated with hot air, place a filter over the air registers in each room.

Install a humidifier in your bedroom to keep your air passages moist while you sleep. Also investigate the benefits of using a room air filter (see "Air Filters for Easy Breathing" on page 22).

In addition to using these appliances, you can help your lungs by changing the way you houseclean. Start by throwing away your broom. Scattered dust from sweeping makes extra work for your lungs. Use a mop or a vacuum cleaner instead. They do a better cleaning job; a water-trap model of vacuum is especially good.

Along with the broom, junk unnecessary chemicals that can irritate your air passages. Many are found in common cleaning products. Wash floors with borax instead of ammonia-based detergents. Polish furniture with olive oil, beeswax or a combination. Clean windows with a teaspoon of white vinegar mixed with a cup of warm water (spray it through a plant mister). Freshen the air with a box of baking soda.

EXERCISE AND BETTER BREATHING

When you walk up stairs, do you feel like you're climbing Mt. Everest? Many people with advanced lung disease are convinced they need a mountaineer's stamina just to get around.

If exertion steals your wind, it's tempting to give up strenuous movement. Yet less exercise soon causes breathlessness, too. This vicious circle can lead to a state of total inactivity.

Such unnecessary invalidism saddens Ann Davis, M.D., director

Hot Chili Eases C.O.L.D.

Chili pepper doesn't just make food taste spicier. It's also a centuries-old medicine for bronchitis. Chili pepper contains a chemical called capsaicin that thins mucus and decreases coughing, says California physician Irwin Ziment, M.D.

of the Emphysema Clinic at Bellevue Medical Center in New York. Says Dr. Davis: "I've seen people with the same level of pulmonary function behave quite differently. Some people fight the same disease while others give in to it and complain. Attitude seems to make the difference."

When air hunger threatens you 24 hours a day, it can lead to a sense of panic. But breathlessness is not in itself dangerous unless it is associated with other problems that need immediate attention. Oxygen starvation is a legitimate fear, but it is quite separate from breathing with difficulty, and the two should not be confused. While those with respiratory disease may have to labor to draw sufficient oxygen into the body, the oxygen *does* get where it's needed. If you want to reassure yourself, Dr. Davis suggests that you ask your doctor to order an inexpensive test called ear oximetry, available at some hospital laboratories. The test will reveal whether enough oxygen is getting to your blood cells, and may be all the reassurance you need to stretch your exercise tolerance. Soon you'll find your confidence beginning to bloom.

Another way to exercise more easily is to learn to breathe efficiently. Many people start their exercise program by becoming aware of breath control. The following techniques can make you an expert. Why not give them a try?

- Learn to breathe in cooperation with your diaphragm (see the instructions on this page).
- Breathe through pursed lips to gain greater control. Start by inhaling normally. Then pucker up. Separate your lips just enough to create a tiny air space. Exhale the thinnest, longest stream of air you can. Listen for a gentle whooshing sound.
- Breathe against resistance to build endurance. Lie on your back and place a book on your abdomen. Breathe from the diaphragm. Start with 5 minutes a day and work up to 15 minutes twice daily. You also can gradually increase the amount of resistance.
- Investigate the benefits of hatha yoga deep breathing. Dr. M. K. Tandon, of Repatriation General Hospital in western Australia, working with C.O.L.D. patients aged 52 to 65, discovered that yoga breathing techniques increased the patients' tolerance for exertion, improved their recovery time after exertion, and resulted in greater control over breathing problems. Here's one method you can try on your own. (However, don't do it right after you've eaten. Wait 2 hours after a heavy meal or 1 hour after a snack.)

Wearing loose, comfortable clothing, sit cross-legged on the floor or in a firm, straight-backed chair. Hold your head and back erect but not rigid. Rest your hands, palms up, on your knees or cup them in your lap. Breathing through your nose only, inhale slowly until you reach a feeling of fullness without strain. When your lungs feel comfortably full, pause for 2 or 3 seconds before exhaling slowly and smoothly. Find a rhythm that is comfortable and natural for you. Start your deep breathing program gradually, for a minute or two several times a day, and work up to two 10-minute sessions daily.

Along with learning to breathe efficiently, begin to exercise. If your pleasure is a game of golf, do that. If

For a new twist on breath control, wrap a cloth around your midsection. Holding the ends, pull it snug. Breathing from your diaphragm, tighten the cloth as you exhale and loosen it as you inhale. Practice this technique while sitting, then walking. Pause between breaths, however, to prevent dizziness and hyperventilation.

you prefer to work out at home, that's fine, too. You can get great results just by hiking up and down your living room staircase. Put on a record of your favorite music if you like, then walk at your own pace, building up to 1 hour of climbing a day. Be sure to breathe from the diaphragm through pursed lips.

You'll raise your activity level a great deal by means of these little steps. If you prefer, your doctor can help you by developing a specific exercise program tailored to your needs and physical capacity.

SMALL GAINS ADD UP

It takes long-term courage to make the best of a serious breathing disability, but small gains along the way can boost your morale.

Dealing with gas pains, for instance, is a real problem for someone with any lung disease, and it is especially painful with emphysema. But you can ease the internal pressure with activated charcoal capsules, available at pharmacies. Raymond G. Hall, Ph.D., associate professor of physiology at California's Loma Linda University, published his research on this remedy in the *American Journal of Gastroenterology.* He recommends taking three or four capsules every hour until the gas pains subside. For best results, start taking the charcoal right after eating a meal which you suspect may cause gas. It's thought that charcoal works because it adsorbs the bacteria that produce bloating, and at pennies a pill it's a real bargain.

Chest congestion is another major problem for those with C.O.L.D. One natural way to ease mucus congestion is postural drainage (see the instructions on this page). For extra benefit, loosen secretions beforehand by doing diaphragmatic breathing for several minutes in front of a vaporizer.

It's a simple treatment—just like breathing properly, exercising modestly, eating right and keeping your environment free of allergens. But each little step adds up, and soon you've traveled a long way toward good health.

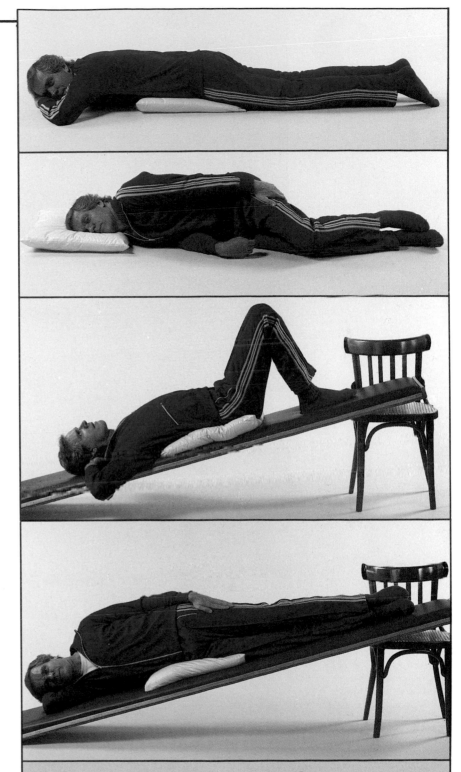

Easing Congestion

The positions shown above, held for 3 minutes each, may be helpful in clearing the lungs. Check with your doctor to see if they will benefit you.
1. Lie face down.
2. Lie on your left side. Swing your uppermost shoulder forward. Repeat on your right side.
3. Using a slant board, lie on your back, arms under head, knees bent.
4. Lie on your left side. Repeat on your right side.
5. Cough vigorously.

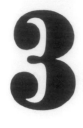

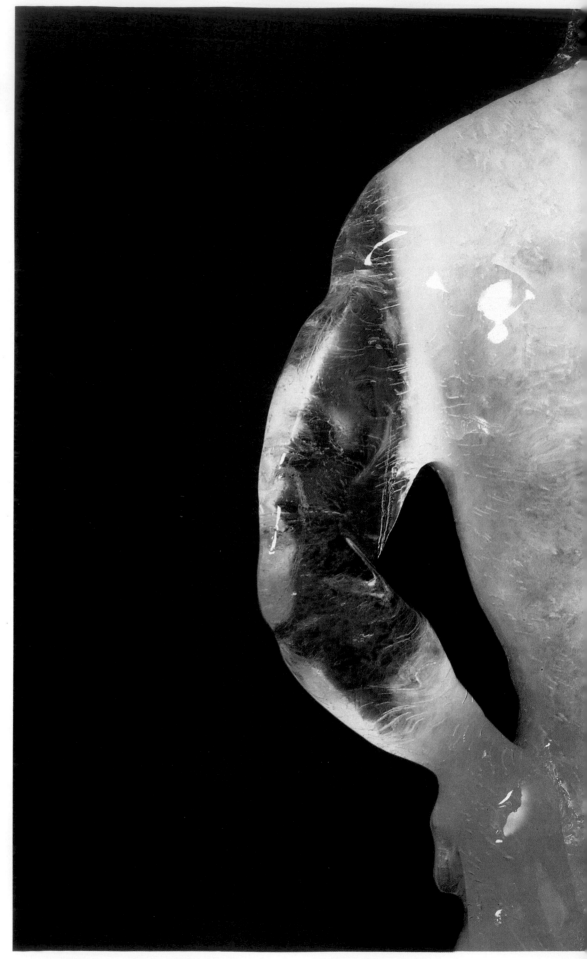

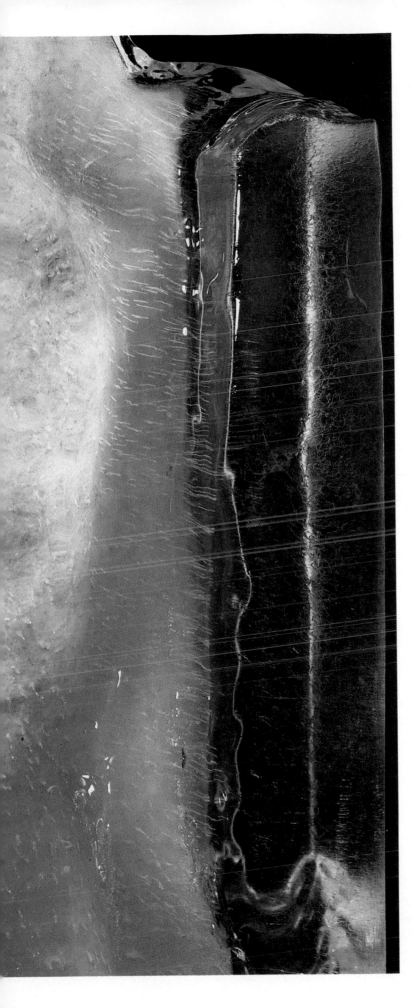

Freeing the Joints

Our bones, joints and spine can retain the fluid grace of youth.

One bone, in and of itself, is not very awe-inspiring. It is a rigid, grayish rod made up of a mixture of collagen, minerals and water. If the body had as its framework just one of these, with our flesh hung like clothes on a rod, we would be capable of doing very little.

Yet take 206 bones, hinge them to each other with intricately designed joints and hook them to muscles by tiny cords known as tendons. Suddenly you have a symphony of parts capable of everything from climbing a mountain to sewing on a button. But, as with a symphony, one note awry or one instrument out of tune can throw the whole performance off. That's exactly what happens with diseases of the bone and the skeletal system.

Consider these, all disorders of the skeletal structure but manifesting themselves in very different ways:

- Arthritis, a mystery illness that afflicts one out of every seven Americans;
- Gout, a disease with a medieval image but a modern-day prevalence: An estimated 1.6 million Americans have this form of arthritis;
- Osteoporosis, a condition that's epidemic among older Americans, especially women, in which the bones become brittle and thin due to a lack of calcium, and which is believed to be preventable, largely by consuming enough calcium;
- Osteomalacia, a disease of bone and muscle weakness due to a lack of vitamin D;
- Systemic lupus erythematosus, a disease of the body's connective tissue, or collagen, that attacks primarily women in their childbearing years.

These disorders, plus sports injuries like fractures, change the course of the day for millions of people and have pain as their common element. Yet a health plan utilizing diet, specific nutrients, exercise and—most of all—a positive attitude can make a huge difference between major incapacity and minor setback. By learning natural treatments, you can keep the symphony of parts that come together as your skeletal system humming for life.

WAYS TO EASE OSTEOARTHRITIS

The trophies stood on the mantel, the frozen metallic figures atop them reflecting what had happened to Don himself. As he looked at them, images slid into his mind: those breezy days in the crew boats on the Charles River. He could see himself reaching forward, putting the oar into the water. Muscles rippling, his limbs working together like the levers of an efficient machine, he pulled back and the boat surged forward.

But no more. Now, when Don awakes in the morning, his body feels as rigid as the box spring below his mattress. At times, the shooting pains in his back and spine are so excruciating that he has to crawl up a single flight of steps. Yet, Don knows that sitting still is the one sure way to give in to his affliction.

Don and some 16 million Americans like him have osteoarthritis, the most common form of arthritis and one marked by pain and stiffness of the joints. It usually is diagnosed after age 50, and can occur in any joint. Men often get it in their hips, while women commonly get it in their hands. Joints that have been especially stressed or injured may be struck with it, such as the knees of an overweight person or the shoulder of a former baseball player.

DAILY UPS AND DOWNS

Although osteoarthritis will become its victim's constant companion, it never becomes chummy enough to be predictable. Helen Faelten, a 65-year-old New Englander, knows of its abrupt comings and goings. One day, she says, she can walk easily, despite a slight pain in her hip. But the next day, she says, she is suddenly "in agony" and can walk only slowly, with a limp.

"I try to ignore this as best I can," says Helen. "When it gets to the point where the pain becomes incapacitating, that's when it really drives me nutty."

Despite its various causes and manifestations, osteoarthritis has one constant element: pain. Many folks toss it off as the expected consequence of getting old, but only the victims know how badly arthritis hurts. Helen says, "Once, after having surgery, I had to hang onto the walls to walk and I couldn't get anyone to understand my agony."

To know how osteoarthritis strikes, it is necessary to visualize how the joints work. In a joint, two bones meet inside a capsule containing a thick "lubricant" called synovial fluid. The end of each bone is covered by a smooth, elastic layer called cartilage. In osteoarthritis, the cartilage has become worn, like the lining of a long-used brake. The bones no longer move easily together; instead, the frayed surfaces grate on each other. Bits of cartilage may even break off and float in the fluid surrounding the joint. It produces

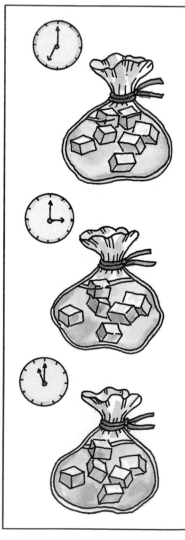

How to Bag the Pain

If heat treatment for your arthritic joints is leaving you cold, try this remedy, used by doctors at a hospital in Philadelphia—ice and a plastic bag!

Here's how it works: Using 2 large plastic bags, fill each with 6 ice cubes and a quart of cold water. Put one on top of your sore joint and the other below. Tightly wrap a towel around the whole thing and relax for 20 minutes. Do this 3 times a day, evenly spacing the treatments.

Twenty-four patients with rheumatoid arthritis tried this treatment for 4 weeks. All said they had less pain even in joints that weren't iced. They found they could sleep better and stand up faster, too.

the same kind of pain you'd feel if you had tiny pebbles in your shoe. In some instances, the body compensates for the deteriorating cartilage by depositing extra calcium at the outer end of the bone. These deposits are most visible when they form in the finger joints, and are so common—especially among women—they've earned their own name: Heberden's nodes.

For most people, osteoarthritis never becomes very severe. The delicate threshold that separates a few aches and pains from osteoarthritis can be recognized by several signs: if a joint has been painful for more than a month or so; if a joint stiffens after a long rest, feels hot or swollen or makes grinding or popping noises when moved; or if small bumps appear at the end joints of one or more fingers.

In making a diagnosis of osteoarthritis, doctors usually depend not only on a physical examination but also on X rays or perhaps an examination of fluid drawn from a sore joint.

BE A FIGHTER

Osteoarthritis is chronic, which means, simply put, that it will almost surely never leave. That thought probably discourages victims as much as their pain. Yet, one part of the body remains untouched by osteoarthritis—the mind, and it is that over which you have control.

Steve Pickert, M.D., who has treated many arthritis victims as a family practitioner in Thurmont, Maryland, says your frame of mind can affect the amount of pain you feel.

"A lot depends on your perception of pain. Your emotional reaction to chronic illness will not make your arthritis worse—but it will make your life worse," he says.

Yet the *best* form of relief for those suffering from osteoarthritis lies literally within arm's reach, although it is not a pill bottle. It's exercise, which, unlike pills that only mask the pain, actually improves the joints themselves. Dr. Pickert says the mainstay of his nondrug approach to arthritis treatment is getting his

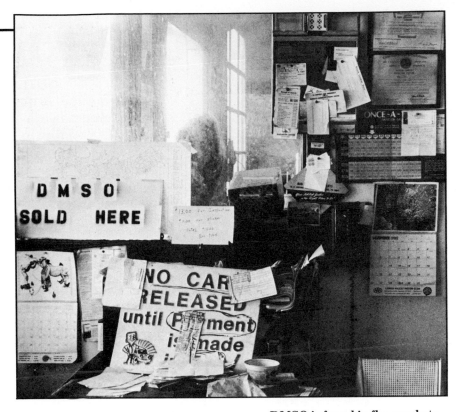

patients to incorporate a balance of exercise and rest.

Exercise has a threefold benefit. First, joint cartilage, unlike other body tissues, has no arteries to deliver nutrients to it. Instead, it is nourished by synovial fluid, which moves through the joints only during exercise. Second, exercise keeps the joints from freezing up. And third, exercise simply gives you a sense of accomplishment.

MOVE YOUR BONES

Exercise may not be easy at first, and that's why it is important to begin at a low but consistent level. Exercise should be done daily. Set aside a "be good to my joints" time, and be sure to choose an exercise that will be fun.

Basically, the exercise should focus on three goals—improving mobility through stretching or range-of-motion exercises; strengthening muscles to make them more stable and better able to bear weight; and achieving overall fitness.

And the exercise does not have to be elaborate. For example, a physical therapist from Washington, D.C., Carol Lewis, has developed an exercise for patients with arthritis of the knee that is so simple it can be
(continued on page 38)

DMSO is found in flea markets, gas stations and veterinarians' offices, but *not* in physicians' and pharmacists' cabinets. The letters stand for dimethyl sulfoxide, a paint thinner. After a chemist inadvertently found it soothed his sore hands, it became publicized as a folk remedy for arthritis swelling. How safe is it? Who knows. Its purity is unregulated and it comes in various strengths—some strong enough to burn or smart. Other side effects range from gorillalike bad breath to the more serious dangers of carrying toxic materials from the skin into the bloodstream and even to liver damage. Tests of DMSO for medicinal purposes have begun. Until they are finished, you'd better apply DMSO to your paint brushes, not your joints.

Loosening Up with Exercise

One-Two-Three Finger Exercise

This exercise will aid in touching fingers to the palm. Begin with the joint closest to the tip of the finger; then bend the knuckle joint, using the other hand to assist.

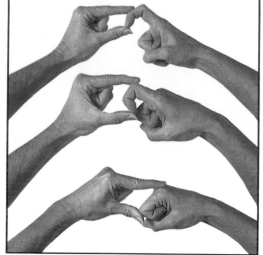

Sitting still is one of the surest ways to let arthritis overcome your joints. On the other hand, exercise can help you regain strength and flexibility. It may mean a little discomfort while you go through a short workout, but the long-term payoff will be worth it. Moving the joints in even the simplest exercises prevents them from freezing up and staves off further muscle degeneration. (Be careful, however, because if pain persists for 2 hours or more after a workout, you've pushed too hard.) Here are exercises that could spell relief.

The Elbow Chop

While seated in a chair, clasp your hands together and bend both elbows until your hands touch your left shoulder, as if preparing to chop wood. Bring your hands down to touch your right knee, straightening your elbows completely. Coax your elbow a little farther than it wants to go. Reverse directions and try again.

The Pendulum

Try these moves to ease a painful shoulder. While standing or sitting, lean forward. Let your arm hang freely in front

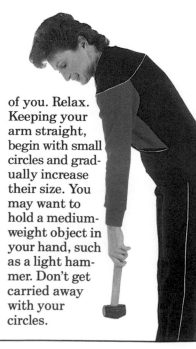

of you. Relax. Keeping your arm straight, begin with small circles and gradually increase their size. You may want to hold a medium-weight object in your hand, such as a light hammer. Don't get carried away with your circles.

The Knee Straightener

This exercise is designed to stretch the knee with a minimum of stress on the joints. Sitting in a straight-backed chair, place your foot on a chair or high footstool. Bend the knee slightly and then straighten your leg by pushing the back of your knee toward the floor.

The Palm Press

Clasp your hands together, palms touching and elbows bent. Press your right hand backward with your left hand, then reverse and press your left hand backward with your right hand.

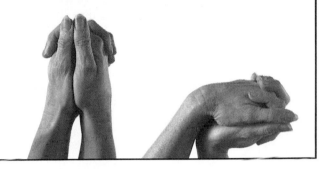

The Foot Roll

Place a dowel (large mop handle, closet rod, rolling pin) under the arch of your foot and roll it back and forth. This feels great and it stretches the ligaments in the arch of the foot.

The Three-Way Neck Stretch

Slowly drop your chin to your chest, then slowly raise your head and gently drop your head backward. Do not proceed farther backward if you feel a sharp pain. Return your head to the upright position slowly. Turn to look over your right shoulder, then turn to look as far over your left shoulder as possible. Tilt your head to the left, then to the right, trying to touch each our to your shoulder.

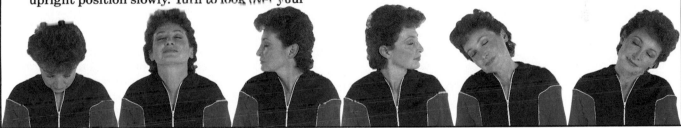

The Pelvic Tilt

This is for the person with low back problems. Lie on a bed or floor with knees bent, feet flat. Place your hands on your abdomen. Flatten the small of your back against the bed or the floor by tightening your buttocks and pulling in your stomach. Think of it as bringing your pubic bone toward your chin.

Knee-To-Chest

This exercise increases the hip motion forward and also helps the lower back. Lie on your back. Keep one leg straight and bring your other knee toward your chest. You can place your hands under your thigh to assist with the stretch. If this is too difficult, start with the other leg slightly bent.

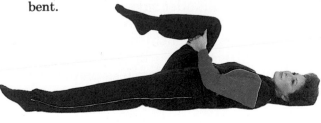

done while watching TV. Just put your foot on an empty bottle and roll it back and forth on the floor, stretching your foot as far as possible.

Never use painkillers while you are exercising, since they might mask your pain and inadvertently lead to pushing a joint too hard.

NATURAL WAYS TO COOL RHEUMATOID ARTHRITIS

It is just a tiny sac surrounding the joint and lubricating it with the body's own oil. But when, without explanation, the synovial membrane suddenly becomes inflamed, it doesn't affect just the joint it protects, but makes the entire body ache and feel tired, stiff and feverish.

That is precisely what happens in rheumatoid arthritis (RA), one of the most common and most disabling forms of arthritis. Three out of four times, its victims are women, although no one knows why. Unlike osteoarthritis, it strikes the relatively young, most commonly those between 25 and 50. Many of the 6.5 million Americans who have RA are in the prime of their lives and have to learn to live with RA's own mysterious clock of good and bad days.

Thankfully, RA is not the end of the line for the great majority. About 20 percent of those with RA recover completely. Most others will experience frequent—even daily—flare-ups of joint pain and swelling, along with flulike symptoms and fatigue. Often, the aching is worse in the mornings but subsides later in the day. For about one in five RA victims, however, the disease will cause permanent joint damage or deformity.

THE INNER WORKINGS

The cause of all this trouble is a tiny body part—the synovial membrane. When this membrane suddenly becomes inflamed, it swells and thickens, as defender cells from the immune system come into it. This inflammation increases the blood flow, making the joint hot as well as swollen.

At a worse level, the defender cells release an enzyme into the joint capsule. The enzyme, normally released to fight foreign bacteria, is strong enough to start eating away parts of the bone. Fortunately, this process doesn't develop for years, which means it can be halted with early medical attention.

Usually, the signs of rheumatoid arthritis are pain and stiffness upon arising; pain, tenderness or swelling in one or more joints, lasting at least six weeks, and recurring pain in the neck, lower back, knees and other joints. To diagnose the disease doctors often depend on blood tests, or they may look for rheumatoid

Pain—A Sure Sign of Rain

How many times have you heard a friend warn that a storm was brewing when there seemed to be nary a cloud in the sky? Then suddenly, out of the blue, a downpour hits.

If your friend is not a weatherman, then chances are he has rheumatoid arthritis.

The old wives' tale that people with RA can predict foul weather is true. A leading doctor of rheumatology, Joseph Lee Hollander, M.D., conducted a study at the University of Pennsylvania Hospital in Philadelphia using a special chamber where weather could be controlled. Patients staying in the "Climatron" experienced more pain when the humidity increased and barometric pressure dropped—the same conditions that happen before a storm. In fact, 73 percent of them had worsening symptoms.

Dr. Hollander says diseased tissue simply does not react as quickly and as well to changing conditions as healthy tissue. Those living in a warm, dry climate will experience fewer barometric changes, and therefore less pain, but moving to the desert doesn't cure arthritis.

nodules, which are lumps, usually the size of a pea, beneath the skin.

Theories about the cause range from blaming a dietary deficiency or a one-celled organism to pointing a finger at the body's immune system. Many experts believe a malfunction in this system is the most likely cause, setting the cells that usually defend the body against the joint itself.

If rheumatoid arthritis is a life sentence, or even a ten-year term, however, many doctors and nutritionists are increasingly finding that much can be done to limit the damage the disease causes, or even limit the disease itself. And it may be nearly as simple as saying, "Hold the mayo!"

A LOW-FAT DIET GETS RESULTS

The Arthritis Foundation has disclaimed, in a practically carved-in-stone message that appears in the literature it distributes, that there is any connection between diet and arthritis.

That is the opposite of what two doctors at Wayne State University in Detroit, Michigan, found. While working with overweight patients, Lawrence Power, M.D., and his colleague, Charles Lucas, M.D., inadvertently discovered that a low-fat diet helped rheumatoid arthritis.

Two of their group had RA, but five days after going on the low-fat diet, their symptoms disappeared.

When one of the patients returned to her usual diet, the pain and swelling came back to her hands. The doctors next tried the same low-fat diet with six other RA patients and got the same good results. Nearly all remained free of symptoms as long as they stayed on the diet.

Yet another researcher discovered that a sensitivity to certain foods can set the joints aflame.

Dan O'Banion, Ph.D., became vitally interested in how foods could throw the body askew not only because he treats many arthritis patients in his psychology practice, but also because he had RA himself. He systematically varied foods, and removed some from his diet. By doing so, he found that apples and also the city water he drank caused

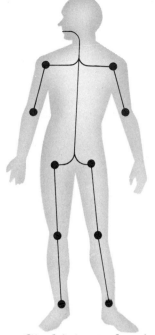

Zapping RA with Zinc

An often underrated player in the mineral world— zinc—may have a place in helping people with rheumatoid arthritis.

Peter Simkin, M.D., found in a study at the University of Washington, Seattle, that treatment of RA patients helped reduce joint pain, swelling and stiffness. In a 12-week study, Dr. Simkin gave zinc to one group and a placebo (a fake pill) to the other. Those taking zinc began to feel much better and their joint swelling went down. The doctor theorizes that low zinc levels cause RA to worsen. Five years after Dr. Simkin's study, similar benefits with zinc were discovered by doctors at the University of Copenhagen, Denmark. They reported that people with psoriatic arthritis, who have troublesome skin problems combined with joint pain and swelling, experienced far less inflammation after taking zinc.

Unfortunately, the flip side is that many folks may not get enough zinc in the first place. Studies analyzing the diets of groups of both old and young people revealed that they consumed one-third to two-thirds less zinc than they need to stay well.

his arthritis to flare.

In a three-month study of three patients, in which he strictly varied their diets by alternating "reactive" and "nonreactive" foods, Dr. O'Banion similarly found that specific foods prompted painful rheumatoid arthritis episodes.

As a result of such dietary manipulation, a 21-year-old woman who had suffered from RA for 7 years found her pain completely disappeared when she ate only fresh fruits, vegetables and fish. Such foods as beef, pork, dairy products and coffee triggered arthritis pain. Dr. O'Banion says the woman remained symptom free even 1½ years afterward, as long as she kept her "reactive" foods to a minimum.

Other researchers are exploring the connection between allergy and

Devices for Arthritics

Shower chairs
Bathtub grab bars
Special scissors
One-hand can
  opener
Clothes buttoner
Velcro hair rollers
Locking pliers
Long-handled
  combs
Key extensions
Raised toilet seats
Book stands
Stocking aids
Chair blocks
Sling towels
Tippers for coffee
Elastic shoelaces

arthritis. In England, 20 out of 22 people with rheumatoid arthritis, following allergen-free diets, found improvement in less than three weeks. Of the 22, 14 learned that grains set off their joints; 8 were sensitive to nuts and seeds and smaller numbers to cheese, eggs, milk, beef and other foods.

The possible link between arthritis and diet traditionally has been given scant attention by the medical establishment. "Most doctors still think of vitamins in terms of the classical deficiency diseases, such as scurvy, beriberi and pellagra. They are not thinking of lesser degrees of symptom-producing vitamin deficiencies that may also impair health," says William Kaufman, M.D., Ph.D.

In Israel, two doctors found that vitamin E apparently provides relief to people with osteoarthritis. In their experiment, I. Machtey, M.D., and L. Ouaknine, M.D., assigned 29 patients—4 men and 25 women—to either a group taking 600 I.U. of vitamin E daily or a group taking a placebo. At the conclusion of the study, 15 of the 29 experienced much less pain while on vitamin E, while only 1 felt better while taking the placebo.

Those who want to pursue nutritional treatments or special diets should inform their doctors of their strategy.

EASING THE PAIN

Few alternatives against arthritis are as "clearly" helpful as water, and it's right at our fingertips. When hot, it increases the blood flow in the joints. If it's cold, it increases muscle tone. A good hydrotherapy program can be achieved with just a bathtub, two deep basins or bowls and an ice bag or ordinary plastic bag (see "How to Bag the Pain" on page 34).

By using a regimen of daily 20- to 30-minute baths, exercise and hot water can help you regain strength and mobility. You can accomplish this by submerging your body in a tub of hot water—100° to 102°F.—and exercising the limbs and joints.

For hands and feet, "contrast baths" have been found to be something of an elixir. By increasing blood flow to the extremities, they help cut down the pain. Begin by filling one basin with cold water (60°F.) and the other with hot (110°F.). Place your hands or feet in the hot water for 10 minutes and then in the cold for 1 minute. Then repeat the process, putting your hands or feet in the hot water for 4 minutes and in the cold for 1 minute. Repeat the 4-minute/1-minute sequence, alternating between the basins six times.

For the arthritic person, daily tasks around the home sometimes can seem impossible. Yet there are ways these tasks can be made easier to do, and there are ways to do them without hurting your joints. One basic principle in joint protection is to use the strongest joint to accomplish a task. The person whose fingers hurt too much to grasp, for instance, may find it easier to open a refrigerator door by placing a strap around the handle of the door, then slipping the forearm through the strap to pull the door open.

Many companies manufacture special devices, clothing, utensils and other items for people with arthritis. A list of such companies may be obtained from the Arthritis Foundation, 3400 Peachtree Road, NE, Atlanta, GA 30326.

For many, the fight against arthritis begins in a pill bottle. Americans spend an estimated $1.3 billion yearly for medications for arthritis.

Aspirin remains the preferred treatment, since it can reduce the inflammation of RA and kill pain. But it also causes digestive problems—from sour stomach to vomiting or ulcers—or ringing in the ears and hearing loss. A variety of aspirinlike drugs—called nonsteroidal anti-inflammatory drugs—have been introduced. The most popular of these are Motrin (ibuprofen) and Clinoril (sulindac).

Dr. Steve Pickert advises patients to weigh the benefits versus the risks, and says that for milder, short-term problems, the new drugs may not be necessary. If you must take any medication, take several precautions: Watch for signs of stomach problems, take the lowest possible dosage and always take the pills with meals or a glass of milk.

THE WINNING STRATEGY

Yet, many who suffer with arthritis, like Vivian Askew of Pennsylvania, have discovered there's really only one drug that truly overcomes this disease—big doses of "will power."

"Arthritis can knock you flat. Many days I went on just pure will power," says the 49-year-old woman. First stricken with rheumatoid arthritis when she was 15, Vivian says her shoulders hurt constantly and her hand felt like it was "on fire." Vivian's doctors prescribed a variety of painkilling drugs which did little but make her very nauseated. Tired of taking pills and feeling no better, Vivian says she decided "to do it on my own." She stopped taking medication, began walking up to 5 miles daily and relied on a lot of will power, as she says.

The result: Much of her pain has gone away and she feels great.

Her precise formula may not work for you, but the important thing is that each person with arthritis must have a game plan. The *disease* can control your life or *you* can take charge of it. Medication is just one tiny piece in the jigsaw puzzle comprising arthritis treatment, along with rest, exercise, diet, specific nutrients and most of all, attitude. Arthritis is a tough opponent but you have the right strategy to outsmart it.

GOUT, A MODERN ILL

All that Gene knew when he awoke in the middle of the night was that his whole body felt like a boiling test tube about to explode at his big toe. What he didn't know was that his pains were all oddly linked to an anchovy pizza, a new job and a strange quirk in his body's inner workings.

If you ask someone with arthritis how they've been managing, and they reply, "swimmingly," they just may be hinting about the great new therapy they've found. Swimming helps increase suppleness and strength. Try it at your local Y, health club or gymnasium. In water up to your chest, most of your body weight will be supported for you. If you don't feel like swimming, try walking instead. The key is to simply move in water, bending or stretching. If you have any concerns about trying this technique, check with your doctor beforehand.

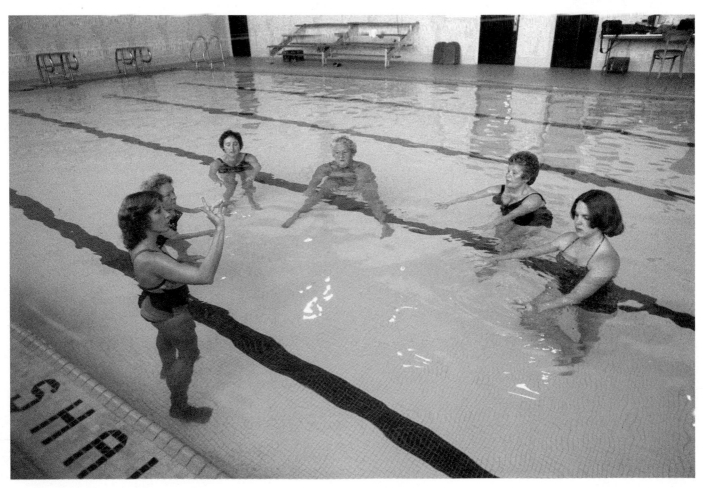

Limping, Gene went to his doctor's office the next morning. There, he found out the bad news—he had gout, a painful kind of arthritis which, despite its medieval image, is very much with us today.

The name "gout" comes from the Latin word *gutta,* or drop, symbolizing the belief during the Middle Ages that it was a disease in which drops of poison slowly inflamed the joints. Instead of being caused by drops, gout stems from crystals of excess uric acid, a waste product of the body, which get into the little space in the joint between the ends of the bones. Imagine squeezing splinters of glass between your thumb and forefinger, and you'll get a fair idea of the pain involved.

Gene, a 47-year-old division manager in a large retail store chain, personifies many of the 1.6 million persons in the United States who suffer with gout. He is typical first of all because gout strikes middle-aged men far more often than women. Second, in the week prior to his attack, Gene had begun his new pressure-filled job as division manager. In supervising new store openings, he felt a lot of stress trying to get architects, builders, landscapers, wholesalers and store employees to work on the same timetable. Trying to forget the week's pressures, he

treated himself one night to a large anchovy-topped pizza, washing it down with Chianti. He might as well have splashed lighter fluid over his joints and struck a match. Both diet—especially foods that contain certain substances—and emotional upsets can spur gout attacks. While the inborn factor that causes gout is usually inherited, the disease is also largely one of lifestyle.

NOT ONLY KINGS AND POETS

It actually can lie dormant long before any attack occurs, as the body collects an elevated level of uric acid in the blood. This acid is usually carried to the kidneys, where a portion of it is eliminated. But due to an inborn error in metabolism, the body of a person with gout either produces too much uric acid or does not excrete enough of it.

Gout's first stage, which is simply having an elevated level of uric acid, is known as hyperuricemia. The person with hyperuricemia may go along, quite unknowingly, until the uric acid is so dense that it begins to form crystals. Then suddenly—often in the middle of the night—gout attacks the joints. In three out of four cases, it first hits the big toe. The stricken joint becomes red, swollen, aching and so tender that even the slightest movement or the weight of a bed-sheet prompts pain. The disease can also affect the knee, the ankle, the instep of the foot, or less frequently, the shoulder or elbow. Gout's only blessing is that it has a narrow focus, almost always striking one joint at a time. In rare situations, two, three or four joints may be affected.

The attacks usually last from about 3 to 11 days, after which the joint returns to normal. About half of those who have an attack never have a second, but for the rest, it becomes a recurring, painful visitor.

At its worst stages, gout is no longer intermittent but becomes chronic, causing deposits of chalky material—actually made up of uric acid crystals—called tophi. The tophi form around the joints or on the ears, and can be removed surgically.

Gout has long been the curse of man—a curse without an effective treatment. This artwork from the early 1800s reflects the usual remedy—bandage your foot and elevate it—as well as the usual result—continued pain. Fortunately, today we know what causes the disease and how to control it with diet.

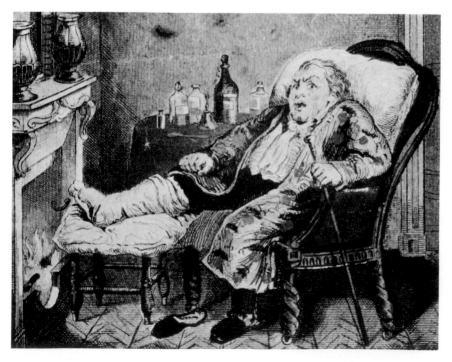

PURINES ADD UP

It's no accident if an anchovy pizza, a snack of sardines or a rich beef dinner set off an attack of gout. While diet is not the cause of gout, it does play a major role. Medical researchers have found that gout is often aggravated by foods that are rich in purines. These are complex compounds which, in breaking down, form uric acid as a waste product. Eating purine-rich foods is like loading up a funnel, forcing the body to break down and eliminate excess purines. The result is an overload of uric acid.

Purine-rich foods include organ meats, sardines and anchovies, gravies and mussels. When the native Maoris of New Zealand left their usual fish and vegetable diet for beef, dairy products, sugary goodies and lamb, they not only became overweight and prone to heart disease but also developed numerous cases of gout.

Alcohol was long suspect as a factor in gout attacks, but the actual connection was not traced until the 1960s by a researcher in Pittsburgh. Gerald Rodnan, M.D., conducted a study at the Presbyterian University Hospital to see if alcohol has any effect when taken with a purine-rich meal. The answer: It sure does. After stabilizing the uric acid levels of six men and one woman, Dr. Rodnan gave them a large evening meal containing purine-rich foods. When the meals were eaten without alcohol, the uric acid levels rose a bit, but when the patients consumed alcohol, the levels jumped markedly. Six of the seven patients experienced gout attacks within the next four days.

NO MANHATTAN— JUST THE CHERRY

Fortunately, the disease that evokes an image of Henry VIII writhing in pain for many long years now can be halted before it becomes chronic. The first step is corraling one's lifestyle by losing weight, limiting high-purine foods, drinking lots of fluids to help get the uric acid out of your system and cutting back on

---

Guidelines for a Low-Purine Diet

TO AVOID GOUT, AVOID THESE FOODS

Approximate purine content ranges from 150 to 1,000 milligrams each per 3½-ounce serving.

Anchovies	Heart	Mincemeat
Asparagus	Herring	Mushrooms
Brains	Kidney	Mussels
Consommé	Liver	Sardines
Gravies	Meat extracts	Sweetbreads

TO AVOID GOUT, LIMIT THESE FOODS

Approximate purine content ranges from 50 to 150 milligrams each per 3½-ounce serving.

Beans, dried	Oatmeal	Whole grain
Cauliflower	Peas, dried	cereals
Fish	Poultry	Yeast
Lentils	Seafood	
Meats	Spinach	

---

alcohol. Also, doctors can prescribe medicine to block the inflammation.

Some gout sufferers have literally found a sweet ending to their gout—eating cherries. The folk remedy was first described by Ludwig Blau, Ph.D., in the late 1940s. Dr. Blau, nursing a severe case of gout, stumbled upon the cherry remedy after nibbling a bowl of the little red fruits and noticing that his gout pain vanished. So long as he ate cherries, his pain stayed away.

Readers have reported to *Prevention* magazine that cherries helped their gout, too. A Nebraska woman wrote that her husband, after trying painkillers and other drugs, got relief after two days when he ate cherries. Those who ate cherries say canned, fresh and frozen cherries— and even cherry juice concentrate— all have helped.

KEEPING BONES STRONG

Bones, as body parts go, do not outwardly demand a lot of attention. For years, decades even, they go

It's Never Too Late to Strengthen Your Bones

Researchers at Kentucky State University concluded that supplementing the diet of elderly women with calcium-rich foods such as milk and calcium capsules built up their thin bones "in a relatively short period of time." Twenty women, whose average age was 70 and who all had osteoporosis, were given 2.25 ounces of cheese and three capsules, each containing calcium, phosphorus and vitamin D, daily. At the end of 6 months, the average bone density of the group increased by approximately 11 percent. Although every individual did not have thicker bones at the study's conclusion, more than half of the women had experienced a significant increase.

about their business of carrying the body's load. But don't let this unobtrusive quality fool you. Little by little, from as early as age 25, the bones are literally sapped of the substance that gives them strength.

Quite unexpectedly, after 30 or 40 years of subtle change, the bones break even without being subjected to force, causing falls and even death, or they curve like the spine of a swayback mare, bending under weight and eventually becoming deformed. This loss of bone strength—the result of continued thinning and increased porosity—is known as osteoporosis, one of the most ignored epidemics of our time.

This condition is the single leading cause of disability among all women over the age of 60. Ironically, osteoporosis is also one of the most easily preventable diseases. It results primarily from inadequate calcium intake. By failing to provide sufficient calcium for your body, you allow your bones to wear down until they are lacy, fragile and thin.

THE BROKEN HIP SYNDROME

The sad consequences of bone loss: Irene, an energetic 72-year-old woman from Cape Cod, has, as usual, put together a reunion for her children and grandchildren. But in bounding around as she serves everyone, she suddenly slips and breaks her hip. Her doctor concludes Irene's hip probably broke, and that sent her falling to the ground, rather than vice versa. She is suffering from osteoporosis.

Seventy-seven-year-old Gertrude has not seen her sister for 15 years. Mary, the younger of the two, instantly recognizes Gertrude as they meet in the airport, remembering well her sister's bright eyes and infectious smile. But Gertrude seems to have shrunk by 5 inches or so, and her shoulders and back are hunched noticeably. Gertrude has a "dowager's hump," a sign of osteoporosis of the spine.

These are hardly isolated cases. Some 200,000 times per year, the same split-second accident that happened to Irene, when her hip spontaneously broke, is repeated in this country. All told, an estimated 6.5 million Americans suffer from osteoporosis. The disease is four times more common in women than in men, and much rarer in black people than in white.

Osteoporosis results from insufficient stores of calcium. Imagine the body having two "bank accounts" —one for savings, the other for writing checks. In this case, the currency is not greenbacks, but calcium. Now suppose the body keeps spending calcium by writing lots of checks, but never makes any deposits in the savings account. Sooner or later, the body will have insufficient funds.

Instead of a savings account, the body uses the bones and teeth to store all but 1 percent of its calcium. That 1 percent is critical, moving about in the bloodstream to power our muscles, brain and breathing. Whenever more calcium is needed for these functions, it is simply withdrawn from the calcium that's banked in the bones and teeth. As you grow older, there is usually more calcium *withdrawn* than *deposited.* In women, bone mass especially diminishes after menopause, in large part because the body no longer produces estrogen, which aids in retaining calcium for new bone formation. So postmenopausal women are the prime targets for a low calcium balance.

In many ways, calcium—and hence, the health of our bones—has been done in by our changing diet. A U.S. government survey found that between 1965 and 1977, per capita milk consumption decreased for all age groups except those over 65. During the same time, soft drink consumption increased among all groups except men over the age of 75.

The Recommended Dietary Allowance (RDA) for calcium is 800 milligrams per day, but many doctors believe that is barely sufficient to stave off osteoporosis. Robert Heaney, M.D., vice president for health science at Creighton University, Omaha, Nebraska, and an expert on osteoporosis, says children and young adults should consume about 800 to 1,000 milligrams daily. Women after menopause, who are the high-risk group, need 1,200 to 1,700 milligrams each day.

Yet getting adequate calcium is still only part of the road to strong bones. Lack of exercise, lack of sunshine, smoking, caffeine and a diet too high in protein may all serve to negate the calcium reserve of the body. The sunshine vitamin, vitamin D, helps the body to absorb more calcium from the food you eat.

Exercise, too, is a key factor in keeping the bones dense and healthy rather than pocked by holes. A Wisconsin researcher, Everett L. Smith, Ph.D., discovered that a simple three-day-per-week exercise regimen could actually increase bone mineral mass in older women. And the exercise need not be strenuous. In fact, he developed 85 exercises that could be done sitting in a chair.

Protection against osteoporosis is truly a lifelong approach, but an easy, natural one. The "one-two punch" of getting adequate calcium every day and exercising may well mean the difference someday between relishing an active, good life or watching it from the sidelines.

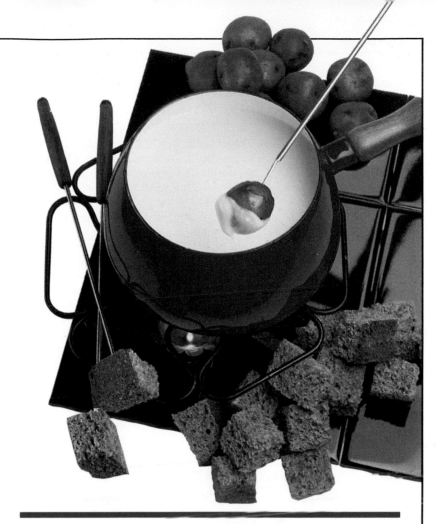

Swiss Goatherds' Fondue

Makes 4 servings

- 1 clove garlic
- 1½ cups apple juice or white grape juice
- 3 tablespoons lemon juice
- 1 pound shredded Swiss, Gruyère or Jarlsberg cheese
- 2 tablespoons whole wheat flour
- pinch of cayenne pepper
- crusty whole grain bread, cut or torn into bite-size pieces and air-dried for a few hours (for dipping)
- tiny new potatoes, steamed and kept warm (for dipping)

Rub the top of a double boiler with garlic, then discard. Pour in apple and lemon juice and heat over simmering water until hot. Toss cheese with flour and add it gradually, stirring constantly to prevent lumping and stringing. (Do not overheat or cheese will form a lump.) When creamy and smooth, like thick white sauce, transfer to fondue pot and keep warm enough so the cheese is melted, but never boiling. Stir in cayenne.

ADULT RICKETS

Ethel's skin was almost a yellowish white, like the color of the corn from the fields she trod as a youngster. But it had not gotten that pale overnight. For more than three years, the 82-year-old woman had not left her house.

Now Ethel was being admitted to the local hospital as a "holiday relief" patient so that the home helper who visited her once a week could take a vacation. There, doctors discovered that the bones in Ethel's chest and shoulders were tender, almost mushy, and her ribs were riddled with tiny fractures.

It was little wonder. Ethel's long-time isolation from the sunshine had led to osteomalacia (adult rickets) a little-known but painful disease. It is marked by a loss of bone density, which causes bones and muscles to be weak, tender and aching. It occurs because of a lack of vitamin D, which helps calcium to be absorbed by the intestinal wall and to be deposited in the bones.

Osteomalacia is very uncommon in the United States. It is a threat, however, to the elderly, especially those living in institutions or who otherwise may not get outdoors often to benefit from the sun's rays. It has been well documented in Great Britain, where fog and rain are the rule.

The hot, streaming sun of the summer months is the best source of vitamin D. In winter, we get a lot less vitamin D from the wan sunlight, especially in northern cities, where the low sun is no match for towering skyscrapers.

Of all the vitamins, vitamin D is one of the more unique. It shows perfectly how our bodies are tied to nature because it is created simply by exposure to sunlight.

Moreover, this vitamin is fat soluble, meaning the body stores it. Therefore a deficiency may not develop until spring.

In winter, then, everyone—especially the elderly—may have to build up their vitamin D stores from food sources. The greatest amounts are found in fish high in oil, such as cod, sardines and herring, and in liver and egg yolks.

Plenty of folks may not get enough of the valuable vitamin from food or the sun, and a dietary supplement may be advisable. In a five-year study of 304 elderly persons in New Mexico, researchers found that 60 percent of those who were not taking supplements had average daily vitamin D intakes of 100 I.U., far below the RDA of 400 I.U. They advised daily supplements to meet the recommended amount. Be careful however, not to exceed the RDA. Too much vitamin D can cause problems of its own.

Winter Sunshine: Boning Up on Vitamin D

The body has no fuel gauge showing whether our exposure to sunlight is enough to keep our vitamin D supply "full" or whether we're running on empty, so deciding whether to take a supplement can be tricky business.

It depends on many factors, especially age and exposure to sunlight. For the elderly, taking a supplement may be necessary. A study of 62 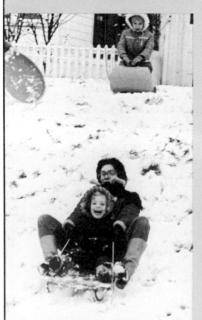 geriatric patients showed that sunlight appeared to have no effect on their vitamin D levels. Yet once they took supplements, their levels went up. For younger people, the opposite may be true. Researchers in England found in a study of 110 children and 11 adults that vitamin D levels were determined more by exposure to the summer sun than by dietary intake of vitamin D. Be mindful that more than 400 I.U. daily of vitamin D is risky.

LUPUS: THE RED WOLF

Imagine a country that is very well protected by an army. Suddenly, for no apparent reason, the army turns on the country itself. Small groups of soldiers, using guerrilla tactics, wage war over the entire countryside, fighting citizens. At times peace returns, but then the army attacks again.

This country is your body; the army is your immune system. A disease called lupus—systemic lupus erythematosus—causes the immune system to turn against the body in the same way that the guerrillas turned against their own country. In lupus, for unknown reasons, antibodies that normally fight against viruses and disease suddenly attack the collagen, the protein substance contained in skin, bones, cartilage and other connective tissue. Lupus can affect the skin (*discoid* lupus erythematosus), or can strike the blood, joints, the central nervous system or the kidneys (*systemic* lupus erythematosus).

None of the estimated 1 million Americans who have lupus could probably tell the same story of their illness. One woman, for instance, may have chest pain, shortness of breath and fatigue, while another experiences aching joints and yet another has a kidney malfunction. Yet there are some similarities. The unique sign of lupus is a "butterfly rash" on the face, experienced by most people with this disease. And, nine out of ten lupus victims are women, primarily in their childbearing years.

Twenty-five years ago, lupus was considered usually fatal, but treatment has improved so dramatically that the majority of those with lupus can lead normal lives. Flare-ups can often be controlled today with long-term cortisone treatment. It has potentially serious side effects, however.

One lupus victim, Betty Hull of Corpus Christi, Texas, was so tired of taking a "shoebox-full of drugs," as she says, that she began her own nutritional fight against lupus 16 years ago. In her case, the disease went into remission and has remained so for 16 years. Thrilled, she started a nonprofit organization, LEANON (LE-Anonymous).

Her nutrition program recommended drinking several glasses of carrot juice a day to ensure a high but safe intake of vitamin A. She also

Lupus—A Disease Named Wolf

Few other diseases leave as unique an imprint on its victims as does systemic lupus erythematosus (SLE). It literally stamps a classic sign on many who have it. Called the "butterfly rash," it involves redness that begins on the bridge of the nose and fans out like butterfly wings on both cheeks.

Rashes such as the butterfly type prompted writers in the 19th century to coin the term "lupus" (Latin for "wolf"), because the rash reminded them of the bite of a wolf. Because of this dramatic symptom, lupus is often thought of as a skin disease. It is not. Rather, it is a disease of the body's inner connective tissue. Like rheumatoid arthritis, one of its sister connective-tissue diseases, lupus is chronic, and attacks far more women than men. The lupus rash may appear as shiny lumps on the facial skin or simple reddening—often popping up after exposure to sunlight.

suggested supplementing the diet with B complex vitamins along with individual B vitamins, including PABA (para-aminobenzoic acid), pantothenate, niacin, choline and B_6. The program was completed with supplements of vitamins C, D and E, as well. She also recommended taking extra calcium.

Later, Mrs. Hull "tapered down" her daily program, she says, to a multivitamin and multimineral supplement, still including, but in lesser amounts, vitamins A, C, D, E and B complex. She takes extra calcium, and B vitamins "as needed." To find out more about LEANON, write to P.O. Box 10, Corpus Christi, TX 78410.

EXERCISE INJURIES

Christine abruptly found out a "natural" law as basic to softball as Newton's law of gravity is to the universe: In a match between knees and spikes, the spikes always win. She was jumping up to catch a fly ball, but just at the moment Christine reached up with her glove, the centerfielder slammed into her. His spikes went into her knee with the force of a sledgehammer.

Embarrassed, Christine shrugged off the throbbing of her knee and kept on playing until the end of the game. She didn't rest, put ice on her knee or elevate it as her teammates urged her to do.

Four hours later, Christine could hardly walk and her knee had swollen to twice its size. Struggling into the car, she drove to the local hospital emergency room.

It was late in the 1980 season when Carl Yastrzemski, the Boston Red Sox all-star outfielder, ran into the right-field wall while attempting to snare a fly ball. Yastrzemski fractured a rib. The injury hurt Yaz so much that he found it tough even to breathe. After a few weeks, Yastrzemski took batting practice but still could not play in a game. He was out for the rest of the season.

As more Americans don track sneakers, smack racquetballs and swim laps in the pursuit of fun,

exercise and competition, more also find sudden, unhappy endings to their exercise. Sports injuries have become perhaps the costliest side effect of America's fitness craze.

About one of every two adult Americans exercises daily, polls show. Unfortunately, the boom has translated into all too many of them being helped off playing fields or wheeled into emergency rooms. Almost 11 million persons are injured in sports each year, according to a special study by the Consumer Product Safety Commission. And government reports indicate the number of sports injuries is increasing by 8 percent each year.

NEEDLESS RISK-TAKING

Yet believing that an injury is the natural consequence of playing a sport is like thinking that a good meal has to lead to indigestion. In Carl Yastrzemski's case, an in-shape, highly trained, professional athlete, in the throes of pennant fever, tried too hard and ran into a wall. However, in a majority of cases, those elements are missing. The victim is not a well-trained professional, there is no major league pennant at stake and the accident is not a freak one. To the contrary, as in Christine's case, people often are injured while playing sports because they overuse or strain a body part, keep playing after they have been hurt, fail to train properly or take needless risks.

You may save yourself from becoming one of the names on a medical log somewhere if you carefully weigh a few considerations before crossing the starting line: What are the safest sports? How can I prevent an injury? What equipment do I need? What kind of training does the sport require and what is the best pace? If I am injured, what should I do?

Richard Dominquez, M.D., chief of surgery at a hospital in Illinois and sports physician for many high school and college teams, advises several steps for the novice about to dive into a sport or regular physical exercise. Dr. Dominquez recommends a weekly schedule of regular

RICE: Sports First Aid Boiled Down

Winning in sports often comes down to minutes and seconds. Likewise, overcoming the most common sports injuries often is determined by how they are treated in the first seconds and minutes after the injury. The staple of immediate first aid treatment is RICE, but it is not a delicious carbohydrate. It's a first aid acronym standing for Rest, Ice, Compression and Elevation, the standard immediate treatment for almost all athletic injuries. It entails these steps:

Rest. Stop using the injured area at once. Continuing may well worsen the damage.

Ice. Application of ice lessens the bleeding from injured blood vessels, thereby speeding the recovery process.

Compression. This limits swelling by impeding the flow of fluid and blood leaking to the damaged area.

Elevation. Elevating the injured part above the level of the heart aids in draining off fluid.

aerobic activity—walking, jogging or swimming—and cautions beginners to start slowly, with perhaps 15 minutes of exercise every other day. If you are over 30 and out of shape, Dr. Dominquez urges a medical examination and clearance from a doctor before huffing and puffing ahead. Once the exercise or sport is begun and you are used to the starting pace, gradually add 5 minutes to your sessions, week by week, until 30 minutes of exercise three or four times a week feels comfortable.

RANKING THE SPORTS

Still, all the good sports medicine advice has not been able to prevent lots of sports injuries from becoming part of our everyday vocabulary, from shinsplints to stress fractures. More than 55 percent of all sports injuries occur in four activities—bicycling, baseball, football and basketball—but no sport or exercise is injury proof. There were, for instance, 2,200 injuries in croquet in 1979, says the Consumer Product Safety Commission report.

Sprains, cuts, bruises and scrapes account for about 60 percent of all sports injuries. Fractures account for less than 20 percent, except in football and skiing, in which they are slightly above 20 percent.

A universal indicator of a sports injury, and one too often ignored, is pain. As sports medicine expert William Southmayd, M.D., notes, "Pain is nature saying that something is wrong. When it talks loudly, listen." People often don't. One 33-year-old woman wrote for advice to a runners' magazine, telling how she had run with pain in her inner shinbone for almost three months before finding out she had a stress fracture. She had been jogging an average of 30 miles weekly on paved roads before a bone scan revealed the source of her pain. (For more on stress fractures, see "When the Bones Say 'I Can't Take It!'" on page 50.)

TRAINING TRICKS

As any good coach knows, the best offense is a good defense, and in

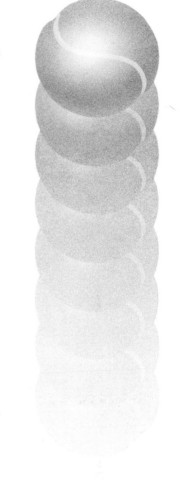

No Tennis Elbow

About half of all those who play tennis daily develop an injury that could easily make them scream louder than John McEnroe does on the court. It's tennis elbow, a painful strain of the forearm muscles and tendons in the joint.

Learning to stroke the right way, by using the entire shoulder and arm, will help prevent this painful injury. When employing a backhand stroke, be sure to distribute its impact by using the entire upper arm. Other factors that cause too much stress on the joints, muscles and tendons include using a racquet that is too heavy or too tightly strung and using heavy tennis balls or a racquet with an improper grip size. Also, don't invite tennis elbow by playing when you are tired.

defending oneself against possible injury, training is the key factor. Begin each exercise session with a warm-up that includes stretching exercises.

Stretching is important in preventing sprains and strains. Any type of vigorous exercise injures the muscle, causing it to shorten and leaving it more susceptible to injury. In stretching, the muscles and tendon areas are lengthened and are made more pliable and less likely to sprain or strain. Such exercises should be aimed at the affected muscles. Bicyclists, for instance, need to stretch their quadriceps—the muscles above the knee—as well as their calf muscles.

Next, get involved in some type of strength training and adapt to any structural abnormalities in your body. Just building up the strength of the muscles through weight lifting may stave off injuries. Studies have shown that strength training makes ligaments and tendons stronger. Also, the bones of weight trained animals have a stronger resistance to fractures, studies indicate.

Never confuse training with overtraining, a phenomenon that happens when you expect to be the Bruce Jenner of the neighborhood with a body that never even heard of the guy. Even professionals do not perform the same heavy workout each day, instead mixing a hard workout with an easy one the next day. Sure signs of overtraining include unexplained redness, swelling, black-and-blue marks, numbness in a limb and no athletic improvement even with rest.

Angus McBryde, Jr., M.D., a Duke University physician who has estimated that more than 60 percent of joggers' injuries stem from training errors, says the best advice a physician can give to a runner is "Listen to your body." That goes for all athletes. Pain is your body's Morse code, and worse injury is invited by ignoring it. You can fake

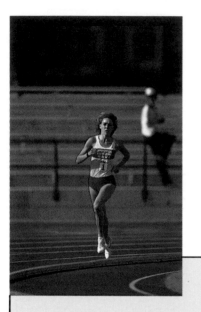

out an opposing pitcher, an attacking lineman, a fellow racer, sometimes even the coach, but you can never fool your body.

STICKS AND STONES...

If, despite careful training, you do sustain an injury—take heart. There's much you can do for even the worst sports injury—the complete fracture. It is considered the most painful of all sports injuries. A bone-breaking tackle, a fall off skates, a ski mishap or any sudden force can cause the bones to snap.

While once a fracture was treated simply by placing the limb in a cast and practically forgetting about it for weeks or months, many physicians are now rethinking the strategy.

"In the old days, they put you in a plaster of paris cast and sent you to bed for a long time. Now we know that may be the worst thing possible," says Jennifer Jowsey, Ph.D., a bone specialist at the University of California at Davis.

Now instead of signing someone's cast, you might want to sign his food shopping list. Researchers have found that the healing of bones can be quickened by feeding the body's increased demands for nutrients.

The body literally starves for protein when a bone is broken, since protein is so critical to new bone formation. Researchers at the Burke Rehabilitation Center in White Plains, New York, found that fracture victims excreted unusually large amounts of nitrogen, an indicator that their bodies were rapidly using up protein. They determined that it would take about 50 days for a patient to catch up with nitrogen losses if he took only the Recommended Dietary Allowance of protein (6 ounces of cod or white chicken meat provide the RDA), but he could cut that figure down to 20 days if he took twice the RDA.

Zinc and vitamin C can also help bones mend, doctors have found. Grant Lawton, M.D., an orthopedic surgeon from Salem, Oregon, tells his fracture patients to take 3 to 4 grams of vitamin C and 50 milligrams of zinc daily.

When the Bones Say "I Can't Take It!"

Stress fractures are the true masked marauders of the sports injury world. They are tiny cracks in the surface of bones, which often can resist diagnosis for weeks or even months. And even though they're tiny, they're mighty when it comes to pain.

Ninety-five percent of all stress fractures occur in the legs and feet. Pain is by far the biggest indicator; nevertheless, it's often tough to detect a stress fracture because the injured bone will respond temporarily to just a couple of days of rest. Stress fractures strike not only the new exerciser, but also serious athletes. Mary Decker, the world-class middle-distance running champion, for instance, was sidelined throughout most of 1974 due to the painful bone cracks. A sure way to detect a stress fracture is by pressing your fingers directly on the painful area, from both above and below. The bone will hurt from both sides. The treatment is straightforward: prolonged rest and then an easy, gradual return to exercise.

Athletic Injuries: Are Females the Weaker Sex?

	Fractures	Dislocations	Severe Sprains and Strains	Extensive Lacerations	Concussions or Skull Fractures	Eye Injuries	Dental Injuries	Tendon Tears	Heat Exhaustion	Cervical Neck Injuries	Total
Basketball	●	●	●	●	●	●			●		7
Volleyball	●	●	●			●					4
Field Hockey	●	●	●	●	●		●				6
Gymnastics	●	●	●		●					●	5
Track and Field	●	●						●			3
Tennis			●			●		●			3
Softball	●	●	●	●	●						5
Lacrosse	●	●	●	●							4
Competition Swimming			●								1
Badminton			●								1
Downhill Skiing			●								1
Cross-Country Skiing			●								1
Fencing				●							1
Bowling			●								1
Soccer			●								1
Synchronized Swimming			●								1
Archery											0
Squash			●								1
Golf			●								1

"We know that zinc and vitamin C are important to wound healing; that's not speculation anymore," says Dr. Lawton.

Exercise may be just as critical to the healing process. Robert Salter, M.D., an orthopedic surgeon at the University of Toronto, believes that immobilizing joints in plaster casts starves the tissues. Based on both animal and human studies, Dr. Salter reported that continuous passive motion (CPM)—moving the joints with a mechanical device through preset movements—aided in healing. The motion helped the synovial fluid to be secreted through the joint, delivering nutrition to the joint cartilage. In one study using laboratory animals, Dr. Salter found that those immobilized in casts showed poor healing after three weeks, and after ten weeks they had stiff joints nearly destroyed by overgrown synovial membrane, the covering around the joint. In contrast, animals receiving the CPM did much better. Half of them began to heal at the end of three weeks.

A COMBINATION OF FACTORS

Almost everyone can avoid painful injuries by following these common-sense steps: Choose your sport carefully, build your body with aerobic exercise and good nutrition, train moderately in your sport and "listen" to your body.

Finally, enjoy your invigorating new sense of health.

Two researchers teamed to examine and subsequently slam-dunk the myth that women athletes might be hurt more easily on the courts and fields than men. After compiling data from 361 colleges and 221 athletic trainers, Christine Haycock, M.D., and Joan Gillette reported that women athletes experienced essentially the same types of injuries in the same numbers as their male counterparts.

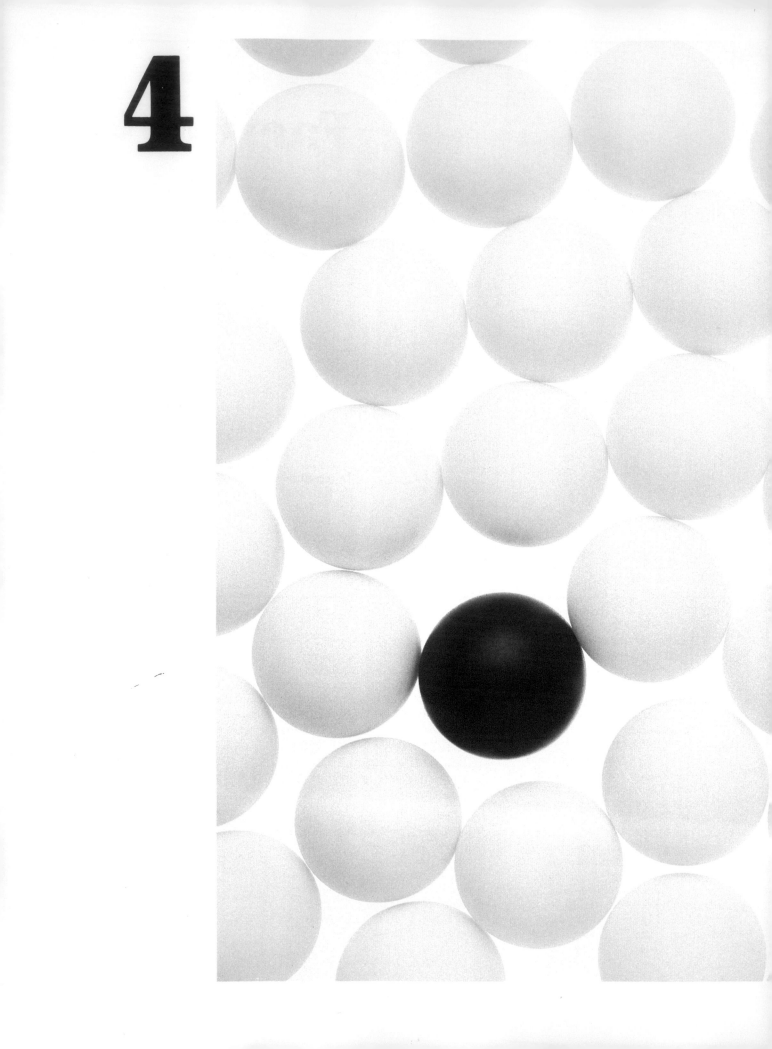

4

Facing the Cancer Challenge

Simple changes in lifestyle and diet may well be our best weapons against the disease.

C ancer may be the most feared word in our language. Uttered by a doctor as a diagnosis, it is received by the patient as a death sentence. But much of our fear is unfounded. In recent years we have learned sure ways to prevent various forms of cancer, and even ways to cure others.

Without a doubt, continuing research will bring us even closer to understanding and curing this dreaded disease.

But cancer is a complex ailment, and one that requires *your* personal scrutiny, as well as that of laboratory scientists. What requires your involvement is this: Cancer does not strike arbitrarily, like the Black Plague, but appears to develop most often in people who fit an increasingly well-defined profile. Certain lifestyles, diets and habits—most notably smoking cigarettes— contribute to the development of this disease. As we learn what these risk factors are, we can eliminate them from our lives.

In addition, scientists have discovered certain factors that are linked to *not developing* cancer— the protective elements. While all the facts are not in yet, there is enough research on hand to support the exciting prospect that we have considerable individual control over this disease. That by eliminating or reducing the factors that place us at risk for cancer, and then by striving to include protective anticancer elements in our lives, we greatly increase our chances of preventing—or possibly surviving—this scourge of modern times.

THE CELL THAT GOES ASTRAY

Cancer is characterized by the uncontrolled growth of cells. Normally, cells reproduce by dividing in an orderly fashion. They reproduce for

53

good, healthy reasons: to provide additional cells for growth and development, to replace those that have died naturally and to repair damaged tissue. But when cells continue dividing beyond the body's normal needs, cell reproduction becomes disorderly. Rather than producing material for growth or repair, the additional cells create a mass of tissue called a tumor. Not all tumors are cancerous. For example, a *benign* tumor does not spread, is noncancerous and can be easily removed. A *malignant* tumor, however, will go on to invade and destroy tissues in its path. In that process, called metastasis, cancer cells spread through the blood and the lymph system, forming new growths, or metastases, at other (often distant) sites of the body.

What causes this crazy replication of cells? Most researchers agree that it usually begins with damage to one cell, which then goes astray. And, in fact, scientists have grown adept at producing cancer in the laboratory by exposing normal cells to various carcinogens (cancer-causing agents). The tar in cigarettes, for example, is capable of damaging a cell to the point where it becomes cancerous. Viruses can produce cancer cells. On occasion, so can estrogen. And asbestos. And saccharin. And various other carcinogens in our environment and workplaces.

In fact, according to Arnold E. Reif, D.Sc., research professor at Boston University School of Medicine, heredity is directly responsible for only "a very small minority of cancers," and most others "are caused by environmental factors." These include exposure to certain chemicals, metals, gases, radiation, certain viruses and estrogen. Some of these environmental factors are simply unavoidable in today's world. But the most dangerous of all is completely under our control. It is tobacco smoking. By far the most damaging chemical pollutant, it causes not only lung cancer but contributes to cancer in many other organs as well. In fact, smoking alone is responsible for one-fourth of all cancers. But scientists also have come to realize that smoking is only part of the story. It's evident now that what we put in our

mouths at mealtime—from childhood on—and also what we *don't* put in, has a profound effect on our body's susceptibility to cancer. Dr. Reif has written, "Surprisingly, the largest gains in protection against cancer, rivaling those reaped by the nonsmoker, promise to come from diet."

Next to quitting cigarettes, then, diet must be regarded as the single most effective tool we have at our disposal to build a defense against cancer.

THE DIET/CANCER LINK

Manipulation of the diet is a vital factor in preventing this disease—and surprisingly simple. Foods fall into general categories—those that have been linked to cancer, those that offer protection against it and those that apparently are neutral. Focusing on foods in the "protector" category, the National Research Council, commissioned by the National Cancer Institute, has developed some basic rules that provide, in a nutshell, dietary guidance against cancer.

- Eat less fatty foods. That advice pertains especially to colon, breast and prostate cancers.
- Eat fruits, vegetables and whole grains daily, especially citrus fruits and those rich in beta-carotene (a forerunner of vitamin A). Taking the rule one step further, we might take care to also include foods that seem to protect against cancer for as-yet-unidentified reasons: oranges, grapefruit, dark green, leafy vegetables, carrots, tomatoes, winter squash, sweet potatoes and cabbage-family vegetables such as cabbage, broccoli and brussels sprouts. In addition, it's believed that foods containing the mineral selenium have a protective effect. Fish and whole grain cereals are good sources.
- Eat very few salt-cured, salt-pickled or smoked foods. These include ham, sausage, hot dogs, smoked fish and bacon, as well as pickled vegetables and meats. Cancers of the stomach and

The Government's Priorities for Tobacco

Of the more than $2.5 billion in revenues the U.S. government receives from the sale of cigarettes and other tobacco products, it spends only about $2 million (less than 0.1 percent) trying to warn Americans of the hazards of smoking. Simultaneously, it spends over $15 million a year providing assistance to tobacco growers.

esophagus are linked to these foods.

- Avoid excessive alcohol, especially along with cigarette smoking. Cancers of the upper GI and respiratory tracts are targeted here.

Bruce N. Ames, Ph.D., inventor of the famous Ames test, which scientists use to detect carcinogens, wrote in *Science* that much of the damage done by carcinogenic foods may come about because of an oxidation reaction within the cell. In the process, an oddball oxygen molecule may damage the cell's genetic makeup. Substances that prevent oxidation—called antioxidants—can counter that damage. Dr. Ames states, "Dietary intake of natural antioxidants could be an important aspect of the body's defense mechanism against these agents." He lists these natural antioxidants we should include in our diet: vitamin E, beta-carotene, selenium, glutathione (an amino acid) and vitamin C.

Some researchers are taking nutrition a step further, and are investigating nutrient therapy in patients who already have cancer.

"The role of dietary factors in the treatment and prevention of cancer is becoming increasingly evident," says Kedar N. Prasad, Ph.D., director of the Center for Vitamins and Cancer Research at the University of Colorado. "It represents a whole new frontier of cancer research."

The day may come when diet therapy is widely recognized as essential, not only to the prevention but also to the treatment of cancer. Some doctors, already deeply involved with nutritional therapy for their cancer patients, supply specific nutrients to them intravenously. Others are exploring the use of detoxifying diets (which allow no alcohol, sugar or caffeine and emphasize whole, fresh foods) with gratifying results.

In addition, some farsighted physicians are helping patients to see that their emotions can play an important part in recovery. The body does not function alone, like a machine, but is utterly sensitive to messages it receives from the mind.

Which Foods Help Prevent Cancer? Which Foods May Promote It?

While research is incomplete, mounting evidence indicates that what you eat may affect your susceptibility to cancer. Some foods seem to help defend against cancer; others appear to promote it. How many of the foods listed below have you eaten in the past week?

Defender Foods	Promoter Foods
Broccoli	Frankfurters
Cauliflower	Bacon
Brussels sprouts	Sausage
Cabbage	Bologna
Turnips or parsnips	Luncheon meats
Carrots	Butter
Tomatoes	Cream
Citrus and other fruits	Sour cream
Sweet potatoes	Cream cheese
Milk	Margarine
Spinach	Mayonnaise
Pumpkin	Sugar
Lettuce or chives	Beverages containing
Leeks or asparagus	saccharin
Parsley	Coffee
Green or red peppers	Alcoholic beverages
Sunflower seeds	
Wheat germ or bran	
Liver	
Whole grains	
Fish	

If you are heavy on "promoters" and light on "defenders," you may want to rethink your diet.

Studies have shown that the way a person reacts to cancer, for example, may help determine whether or not he or she will survive the disease without recurrence. In a five-year study of breast cancer patients at King's College Hospital Medical School in London, doctors found the "scrappers" won out. The women who survived cancer without recurrences were the ones who "had initially reacted to cancer by denial or who had a fighting spirit," whereas the patients who succumbed "had responded with stoic acceptance or feelings of helplessness and hopelessness."

"I can [overcome cancer], I will do it. I won't quit. I won't give up."

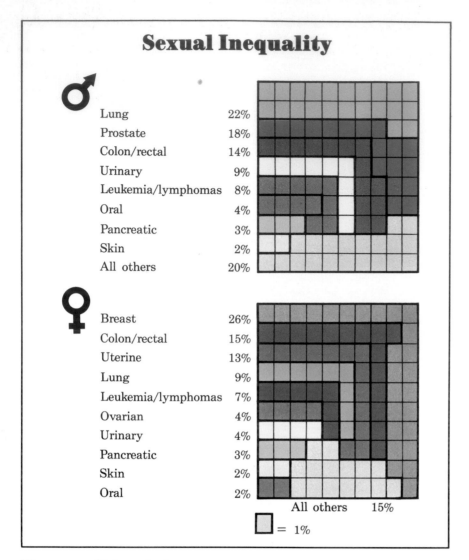

Sexual Inequality

♂

Lung	22%
Prostate	18%
Colon/rectal	14%
Urinary	9%
Leukemia/lymphomas	8%
Oral	4%
Pancreatic	3%
Skin	2%
All others	20%

♀

Breast	26%
Colon/rectal	15%
Uterine	13%
Lung	9%
Leukemia/lymphomas	7%
Ovarian	4%
Urinary	4%
Pancreatic	3%
Skin	2%
Oral	2%

All others 15%

☐ = 1%

Women pay a higher price for being female than men pay for being male, at least when it comes to cancer. The latest estimates show that cancers related to sex organs account for 43 per cent of all cancers among women (breast, uterus and ovary), but only 18 percent among men (prostate). Deaths from these cancers are lopsided, too: 29 percent vs. 10 percent.

These words were echoed and reechoed by cancer patients interviewed for *The Cancer Survivors,* a book by Judith Glassman. Indeed, determination may well be the single common denominator among people who conquer the disease.

And that feeling of determination can be put into use today—not called upon only when you've already become a cancer victim. Using that strong sense of purpose and desire to live fully, root out those habits of diet and lifestyle that can promote the disease. Determine that you can prevent cancer and you will.

LUNG CANCER

Consider this contradiction: Cancer of the lungs is one of the most preventable types. Yet in the last 25

years, it has increased 172 percent among men and a staggering 256 percent among women. And while it is quite easy to prevent, it is quite difficult to cure. It accounts for 35 percent of *all* cancer deaths in men and 17 percent in women.

Cigarette smoking is the single greatest cause of lung cancer. Thus, the single, greatest preventive measure is to quit smoking. Some smokers tell themselves that they've smoked for years and "nothing's happened"—so far. Others keep on smoking, telling themselves the damage has been done; that quitting would make little difference. In fact, quitting at *any* point in life brings improvement. A program for successfully overcoming this dangerous habit appears in chapter 11.

So far we have identified the single most important cause of lung cancer: smoking. But now we should discuss the single most important factor in protecting against lung cancer (other than not smoking): vitamin A.

THE NUTRIENT THAT DEFENDS THE LUNGS

Studies carried out in Norway, the United States, Singapore, England and Japan have all shown that people who have a diet rich in vitamin A tend to have a lower risk of developing lung cancer than people who have a low intake of the vitamin.

If you're at risk, perhaps you should investigate beta-carotene. Studies suggest that getting your vitamin A from beta-carotene gives the *most* protection. Fortunately, it's easily found in many foods and is abundant in carrots, sweet potatoes, collards, winter squash, spinach, kale, broccoli, canteloupe and apricots.

One study, which spanned 19 years, monitored the eating habits and lifestyles of 2,107 middle-aged men at the Western Electric Company in Chicago. Researchers compared that data with rates of cancer, particularly lung cancer, which was diagnosed in 33 men. Of the group who got lung cancer, a full 42 percent were from the group that ate the *least amount* of beta-carotene.

The scientists concluded that cigarette smoking was a significant cause in the development of lung cancer and other diseases. But, they stated, "a diet relatively high in beta-carotene may reduce risk of lung cancer *even among persons who have smoked cigarettes for many years.*"

How does vitamin A work to protect the lungs? The exact mechanism is unclear. But we do know that vitamin A enables the cells that line the lungs, called epithelial cells, to secrete mucus, which bathes the area and keeps it healthy. Cilia, hairlike projections on the lung's epithelium, then help sweep the mucus out of the body.

When there is too little vitamin A in the diet, the epithelial cells lose their ability to form and secrete mucus. They become dry and hard. To add insult to injury, these dry cells lack cilia, so that toxic matter and foreign substances may begin to settle on their undefended surface. And those hardened cells may actually form roadblocks to the openings that allow material to go in and out of the body. In short, due to a lack of vitamin A and the subsequent lack of mucus, these secreting cells gradually lose their ability to protect, and the lungs consequently suffer.

What happens, then, when plenty of vitamin A is available in the body? At all stages of treating lung cancer—including prevention—this little nutrient provided big benefits. For example, French doctors reported that a form of vitamin A helped long-term smokers significantly reduce the magnitude of bronchial metaplasia, a precancerous state of the bronchial tube where the cells have become abnormal. Other studies have shown that even radiation and chemotherapy work better when patients also receive vitamin A. And in a trial involving nine men with a diagnosis of incurable lung cancer, the doctors found that vitamin A used alone—without other therapies—succeeded in stimulating the men's immune response. Giving the patients synthetic forms of vitamin A (vitamin A palmitate or 13-cis vitamin A acid), resulted in a significant increase in cancer-fighting white blood cell activity, which was low before treatment. Vitamin A, however, is a

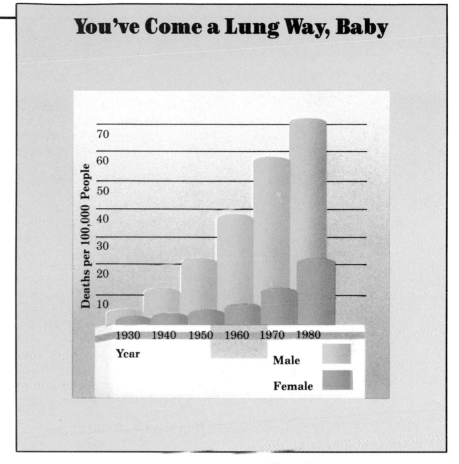

You've Come a Lung Way, Baby

Though lung cancer is more prevalent in men than in women, the rate among women has been rising rapidly. Since 1930, it has increased almost tenfold.

potent substance in high doses, and patients need constant monitoring for toxic reactions.

VITAMINS C AND E ARE ALSO IMPORTANT

Vitamin A is not alone in its role as defender of the airways. Vitamins C and E also seem to provide protection. In fact, according to research from the Louisiana State University School of Medicine, a diet low in these two nutrients may increase the risk of lung cancer. When the diets of 29 people with lung cancer were compared with those of the same number of people without the disease, levels of carotene and vitamins A, C, and E were much lower among those with cancer. And a recent study at a hospital in Leeds, England, showed that lung cancer patients were severely deficient in vitamin C: 64 percent had plasma vitamin C levels *below* the threshold necessary to prevent scurvy. Vitamin C, the researchers said, appeared to be vitally important in stimulating the immune response and repairing tissue.

CANCER-CAUSERS IN THE AIR AND ON THE JOB

To be sure, there are "cancer pockets" across the country, places where the residents face a higher-than-average risk of getting lung cancer either because of air pollution or because of the nature of the industries located in the area. But it is difficult to gauge exactly how much damage air pollution itself causes. Take a city such as Pittsburgh, for example. Heavily industrialized, it's burdened with smog and air pollution. Yet, a study done in and around that city revealed that any differences in the rates of lung cancer there were attributed mainly to differences in smoking habits.

However, exposure to toxins on the job does appear to be a significant risk factor. Asbestos is a prime example. Shipyard workers, construction workers and others who are exposed to it at work have a greatly increased risk of lung cancer and mesothelioma (a type of tumor that develops in the lung). And if they smoke, they increase that risk twentyfold. Because of the interacting effects of smoking and asbestos, this risk could be as much as a hundredfold. Workers in other occupations— miners, foundry workers, gas workers, millers, and more, also have higher rates of lung cancer than the general population.

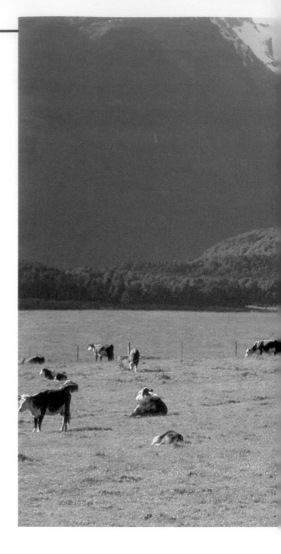

Companies must provide adequate protection, including protective gear for high-risk workers. Use it.

LESSENING THE RISK OF COLON CANCER

Every morning by 7:30, Taro Yamamoto is on his way to work. His breakfast: soup made from soybeans with seaweed, fish, rice, pickled cabbage and green tea. For lunch, he dines at the company cafeteria on buckwheat noodles, steamed spinach with sesame seeds and green tea. He doesn't get home until 9:30, but his wife has dinner waiting for him: an appetizer of raw tuna with horseradish, soup with tofu (bean curd), steamed bamboo shoots, roasted chicken, rice, pickled plums and, of course, green tea.

Taro's cousin Mark lives in Honolulu. He was born in the United States. The Hawaiian Yamamotos

Diet and Colorectal Cancer Linked

A study published in *Cancer* adds new weight to the theory that colorectal cancer is linked to dietary habits. Scientists studying European and American-born Jews living on an Israeli kibbutz discovered a much lower colorectal cancer rate than among their counterparts in Tel Aviv. The researchers concluded that this is probably due to low intake of beef, cholesterol and saturated fat coupled with high consumption of fruits and vegetables providing fiber, vitamins and minerals.

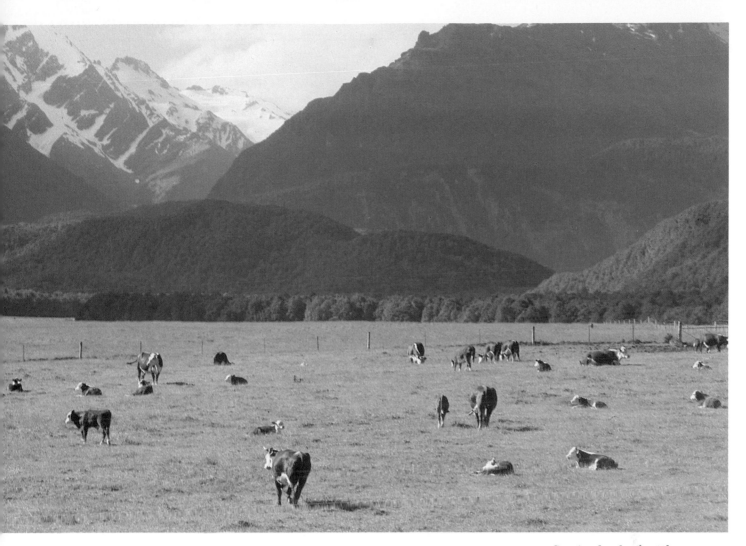

still eat some Japanese foods, but Mark's daily menu reflects just how much his family has adapted to American ways. Mark's favorite breakfast is bacon and eggs— and rice.

Taro and Mark are not real people. But they could be. Let's assume they are both 45 years old and look very much alike, though Mark is a bit taller and weighs more. And now let's assume that we are epidemiologists, scientists who study disease patterns among populations. What do we know about the health of these two men?

Despite a common gene pool, the cousins do *not* have an equal cancer profile. Taro, it turns out, has a low risk of getting cancer of the colon, while Mark, on the other hand, is *four times more likely* to get colon cancer than his cousin.

Mark, you see, lives in the States, where colon and rectal cancer is second only to lung cancer, with an estimated 126,000 new cases each

year; about 58,000 die of it annually. Why?

The reason for this epidemic is probably that we eat too much fat. The American diet averages about 40 percent fat daily, eight times that of Japanese and African diets. Excess fats in the blood stimulate the production of bile acids in the intestine. Bacteria then may metabolize these acids and change them to mutagens—substances capable of altering cells to a cancerous form.

RAISE FIBER, LOWER RISK

If you are concerned about colon cancer, the most obvious protective step you can take is to strictly limit the quantity of meat you eat, along with curtailing the amount of butter, cheese and other fats, especially saturated types, in your diet. You can, however, occasionally enjoy those foods you love, provided you

Grazing herds of cattle are a common sight in New Zealand, one of the few countries in the world where the per capita consumption of beef is higher than in the United States. And New Zealanders also are one of the few groups of people in the world with a higher death rate from colon cancer.

take a second protective step—eat lots and lots of fiber.

Take a lesson from the Finnish people, who eat lots of dairy products and a fair amount of meat. In fact, their diet is moderately high in fat. Yet they suffer little colon cancer. The secret seems to lie in their high intake of dietary fiber. How can fiber-rich foods like fresh fruit, vegetables, whole grains and bran help prevent one of the most devastating diseases of modern civilization? Fiber may work simply by increasing the volume of the stool and thus diluting tumor-causing agents and the concentration of bile acids and bacteria in the intestine. Or it may bind up and evacuate them from the body. Whatever the reason, study after study has shown that a fiber-rich diet helps foil cancer.

In addition to fiber, cabbage and other crucifiers like brussels sprouts and broccoli apparently protect against colon cancer. Healthy people report eating more of these vegetables; colon cancer patients have a history of eating less.

What's remarkable is that not only the vegetables but also the soil in which they're grown can affect our cancer risk. Scientists have found that in areas where the soil is rich in selenium, colon cancer rates are low. Crops grown on such land are high in selenium, and traces appear in drinking water, as well. To find out exactly how effective selenium is as a cancer protector, scientists at the University of Nebraska Medical Center, Omaha, fed one group of rats a very low-selenium diet and another group a high-selenium diet. Then they gave all the rats weekly injections of chemicals that cause tumors. At the end of the trial, the rats on the low-selenium diet had twice as many tumors as the high-selenium group.

VITAMINS C AND E CHALLENGE CANCER

Promising research in nutritional therapy for colon cancer has come from Toronto physician W. Robert Bruce, M.D., Ph.D., who gave volunteers 400 milligrams of vitamin C along with 400 I.U. of vitamin E daily for six months, a regimen which resulted in "significant" reduction in the number of mutagens in their stools.

A Tale of Tucson: Sunny Sky Blues

In recent years, many Americans have abandoned harsh northern winters for the year-round sunshine of the so-called Sun Belt. But while such a move may be beneficial to people suffering from arthritis, acne and psoriasis, evidence linking skin cancer to sun exposure is steadily mounting. Residents of Tucson, Arizona, for instance—a Sun Belt city that boasts the sunniest days, warmest climate and clearest blue skies in the United States—have the highest rate of skin cancer in the country.

By checking records at all 8 Tucson hospitals, Michael M. Schreiber, M.D., and his colleagues at the University of Arizona Health Sciences Center discovered a 340 percent increase in the incidence of malignant melanoma (the worst form of skin cancer) over a 10-year period. In addition, since 1960, the rate of nonmelanotic skin cancers has gone up 500 percent.

Tucson, in fact, is second only to Queensland, Australia—an area of similar sun exposure inhabited by fair-complexioned people (who are more prone to skin cancers than people with more pigmentation)—in the number of residents with malignant melanoma. But you don't need to go to the Sun Belt to run the risk of contracting skin cancer. Anywhere there's sun, there's also risk.

So what can you do about it? "We'd like to be able to convince people not to sit in the sun at all," says Dr. Schreiber. Barring that unlikely prospect, however, he strongly recommends never exposing your skin to the sun without the protection of a sunscreen, especially one that contains para-aminobenzoic acid (PABA) or ester of amino-benzoic acid.

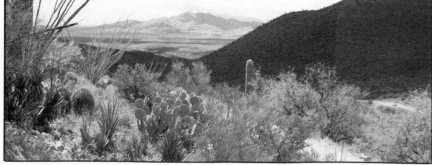

SKIN CANCER, THE MOST PREVENTABLE MALIGNANCY

An estimated 400,000 new cases of skin cancer develop every year in this country. Most are preventable. So say prominent researchers from the National Cancer Institute, the American Cancer Society and the Skin and Cancer Hospital of Philadelphia.

Most people with the problem suffer from nonmelanotic skin cancer. The cause of this disfiguring, potentially deadly disease is deceptively innocent. It's simply staying out in the sun too long. Those most at risk are fair-skinned—people who look like lobsters when they come home from a day at the beach. Americans of Irish, Scottish and Welsh descent suffer the most.

In addition to fair-skinned folk, others likely to suffer from the sun's rays include people who are photosensitive, that is, super-sensitive to sun. Most are especially sensitive because they take certain medications or suffer from diseases such as lupus erythematosus. Those with darker complexions are at less risk, and black people have a very low incidence of skin cancer.

The sun's damage is cumulative; that is, it adds up over time. Consequently, skin cancer occurs more frequently in older people (as is true of most cancers). However, according to researchers at the Temple University School of Medicine in Philadelphia, the middle-aged now are increasingly at risk. It seems our national obsession with sunbathing is at the root of the problem. Karl J. Kramer, M.D., a Miami dermatologist, wrote in the journal *Modern Medicine*, "Although tanning is a protective reaction to sun exposure, it is also *a priori* evidence of sun damage. Put simply, there is really nothing healthy about a 'healthy tan.'"

So, does this mean your sun worshiping days are over? Well, some doctors would say, emphatically, "Yes." But before you sell your farm, give away your sailboat or cancel your trip to Hawaii, there *are* safe ways to enjoy the sun.

First, avoid the most intense ultraviolet radiation by staying indoors between 10 A.M. and 3 P.M. or at least from 11 A.M. to 1 P.M.

Second, use a sunscreen. It can block the most dangerous portion of ultraviolet radiation, the rays called UVB. Thomas B. Fitzpatrick, M.D., of Harvard Medical School, says, "Based on several years of experience using UVB sunscreens . . . the incidence of sun-induced skin cancer is reduced by daily applications of highly effective UVB sunscreens." The lotions that he and many dermatologists recommend contain PABA, a B vitamin that is a natural sunscreen.

RECOGNIZING SKIN CANCER

How can you tell skin cancer when you see it? The answer is not easy, since the disease has many appearances.

Early detection is *vital*, especially when the skin cancer is a less common type called melanoma. This cancer affects the melanocytes, the pigment-producing cells. Often beginning in a mole, it grows quickly and has a much poorer prognosis than that of nonmelanoma.

Melanoma most frequently shows itself by a change in color, a darkening, or an increase in size of a mole or pigmented patch of skin that has been present for years, or from birth. Sometimes a new molelike growth signals cancer. The melanoma may break open and bleed, or appear infected. Aside from solar radiation, genetic factors and some chemicals may play a part in causing melanoma.

Nonmelanotic cancer may appear as a new growth on the skin, perhaps a pale, waxy lump; later, the lump may bleed and crust over. Or the disease may be heralded first by a sore that doesn't heal, or a red, rough, scaly patch that doesn't go away. *Any* unusual growth or sore that doesn't heal should be brought to the attention of your doctor.

If the spot is diagnosed as a malignant *non*melanoma, the most usual treatment is surgery—complete removal of the cancerous area.

If the growth is diagnosed as a *melanoma*, surgery is almost inevitable. However, new and promis-

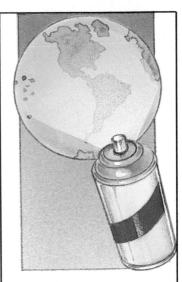

Depleting the Ozone

Even though ozone-depleting chlorofluorocarbons were banned in aerosol sprays, this vital layer is still being eaten away. Ozone acts as a shield against the sun's harmful rays. Scientists predict that the increased exposure to ultraviolet radiation will lead to a rise in the incidence of certain kinds of skin cancer.

ing treatments are being developed. One, called immunotherapy, involves stimulating the body's own defenses to fight the invading cancer. One stimulant used is BCG, a vaccine for tuberculosis.

The other promising therapy relies on vitamin A.

HOPE IN VITAMIN A

Numerous studies suggest that a lack of vitamin A may be associated with epithelial cancers. In addition, animal studies show that vitamin A can "delay tumor appearance, retard tumor growth and regress [epithelial] tumors," says the *Journal of Human Nutrition*. In fact, "Vitamin A and its analogs [derivatives] may have a prophylatic [preventive] and a therapeutic role."

In a study using topical vitamin A treatment, one patient with melanoma had a "complete regression of the treated lesions" and another patient had a "partial response."

In addition, melanoma patients who take oral vitamin A therapy in conjunction with the BCG vaccine have fewer relapses than patients receiving only the vaccine.

A Cancer Detector in a Bra

Can women get help in predicting or detecting breast cancer from wearing a certain kind of bra? An experimental screening device, worn for 15 minutes each month, is reported to have picked up mammary tumors as small as 2 millimeters in diameter in women who had no symptoms. Harold L. Karpman, M.D., an associate professor of medicine at UCLA, said the home tester is being used experimentally as a way to warn women of their increased risk—even those without any symptoms. The device has two plastic-coated aluminum disks containing heat-sensitive dots which change colors to indicate an abnormality in the temperature of breast tissue. If approved by the Food and Drug Administration's Bureau of Medical Devices, the home detection bra would be marketed by a cosmetics firm.

A PLAGUE OF BREAST CANCER

Next time you're in a movie theater, count the number of women seated in the rows in front of you. Stop when you reach 11. If you are a woman, include yourself in that group. One of you will be stricken with breast cancer.

The rate of breast cancer among American women is staggering. Aside from gender, what makes women so very susceptible to this terrible disease? Certain risk factors come into play, some of which we have no control over—a history of breast cancer in the family, beginning menstruation at an early age or never having children. Yet, you can reduce the chance of developing this anguishing disease by focusing on risk factors you *can* control. First is weight control. Scientists have found a link between overweight and breast cancer—especially overweight in postmenopausal women. But equally important is a diet low in fat.

Statistics tell us that wherever there is a lot of fat in the diet, there is also a correspondingly high rate of breast cancer. Japan is a country that has provided a model of how a low-fat diet can keep breast cancer rates low; now, sadly, it is providing a new model. Takeshi Hirayama, M.D., of the National Cancer Center Research Institute in Tokyo, says, "Breast cancer mortality and morbidity rates are on a steady increase in Japan in recent years. Most probably this . . . is the reflection of the increase in the amount of dietary fat intake."

Our standard diet is comprised of about 40 percent fat, and some medical researchers strongly recommend we cut that by almost half. And here are some other suggestions:

Boost Intake of Vitamins A and C. Women seem less likely to develop breast cancer if their diet is rich in these nutrients.

Consume Adequate Iodine and Selenium. Research suggests that a lack of the nutrient iodine leads to abnormal growth of breast cells. Kelp and seafood are rich in iodine. Seafood also contains selenium, a trace metal that seems to protect against breast cancer. Whole grains and Brazil nuts also yield goodly amounts of selenium.

Eat Beans instead of Meat. Beans contain substances called protease inhibitors, which may block the cancer-causing process.

Avoid Coffee, Tea, Cola and Chocolate. These foods contain methylxanthines, substances linked to fibrocystic disease.

Periodic breast self-examination is extremely important. Some 95 percent of all cancerous lumps are discovered at home. And the earlier you detect a trouble spot, the easier it is to treat and/or cure. Radical mastectomy, in which the breast, the lymph nodes under the arm and the chest muscles are removed, is now reserved for very advanced cancers. The modified radical mastectomy is now the standard treatment. This surgery removes the breast and the lymph nodes, but leaves the chest muscles intact. A procedure called lumpectomy removes only the tumor itself, and another therapy designed to preserve the breast, interstitial implant therapy, is being used in some hospitals. After lumpectomy, thin plastic tubes are implanted and radiation is delivered to the site where the tumor was, to avoid recurrence. Radiation and chemotherapy are other treatments.

CANCERS OF THE UTERUS AND OVARIES

"Woman-trouble" is what they called it in the old days. And woman-trouble is what it still is. But those illnesses that develop in the female reproductive organs were far more serious in our grandmothers' time than they are today. Consider this: Since the 1940s, the death rate from cancer of the uterus (cervical and endometrial) has plummeted by more than 70 percent. For a drop in cervical cancer, we have George Papanicolaou, M.D., to thank. His Pap test is now widely used as a screening procedure to tell if a woman's cervical cells are healthy.

For Early Detection, a Step-by-Step Breast Self-Exam

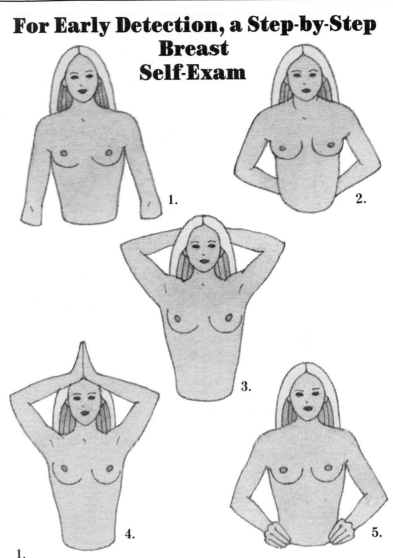

1.
Observe breasts in the mirror for skin pulling, dimpling, nipples scaling or crusting or any watery, yellow, pink or bloody discharge.

2.
Lean forward slightly to observe any changes in the breasts, like skin puckering.

3.
Raise your arms slowly overhead. Examine the breasts for changes.

4.
Then rest your raised hands against your forehead. Observe any changes.

5.
Next, tighten chest and arm muscles. Again look for changes.

Continue the examination by lying on your back with a folded towel under your right shoulder and your right arm tucked around your head. With left hand cupped, use the flat of the fingers to feel for lumps or skin changes in your right breast.

In a rotary direction, examine the inner half of right breast from collarbone to the underportion and from the nipple to the breastbone. Then examine the outer area between the nipple and the armpit (including the armpit itself), where most cancers occur. A ridge of firm tissue in the lower curve of each breast is normal.

Repeat steps; use right hand to feel left breast.

Early detection, as usual, is crucial in controlling cancer.

Endometrial cancer also is on the decline, thanks to a concomitant drop in use of estrogen replacement therapy (ERT) among postmenopausal women. These declining rates are significant and encouraging, yet problems still exist for many women.

The unfortunate statistics are that 99,000 new cases of uterine cancer are detected each year. American women, in fact, are at greater risk of endometrial cancer than British women. Why? Because some older American women are still being treated with straight estrogen—not countered by the hormone progestin—for their postmenopausal problems, while British women tend to take a combination estrogen-progestin pill.

But ERT is only part of the story. As in so many other cancers, obesity and a high-fat diet may make a woman more prone to endometrial cancer. Here's what apparently happens: Excess fat makes the body produce excess estrogen—and too much estrogen has produced tumors in innumerable animal experiments. Other potential risk factors are early onset of menstruation and late menopause (both phenomena are estrogen related), previous cancer of the colon, breast or ovary, high blood pressure, diabetes and infertility. Interestingly, fat may play a role in most of those conditions.

Endometrial cancer most often shows up in women between 55 and 70 years of age. Any woman approaching menopause who recognizes herself in the high-risk profile would be wise to reduce the amount of fats in her diet, lose weight if she's overweight, do all she can to reduce other risk factors within her control (see the chapters on diabetes, heart disease and intestinal ailments), make sure her doctor is well informed of her history and act quickly if *any* symptom of cancer appears.

CERVICAL CANCER AND YOUR DIET

Cervical cancer has a "precancerous" stage where cells are doing strange things but aren't necessarily cancerous. Called cervical dysplasia, this condition is most common in women aged 40 to 60.

Now, doctors are saying that the abnormal cells of cervical dysplasia are sometimes the result of nutrient deficiencies. And that a possible cure for mild to moderate dysplasia may be just a supplement away. Charles

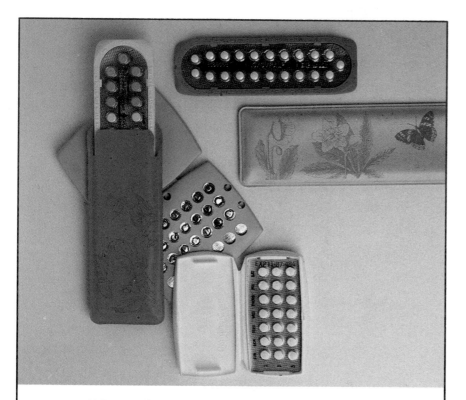

The Pill: More Implications

Is there a link between birth control pills and cancer? Possibly, according to 2 different research groups who reported their findings in *Lancet*, a British medical journal. After a study of 9,992 women, doctors in Oxford concluded that women who use oral contraceptives on a long-term basis may be at a greater risk of getting cervical cancer than women who use intrauterine devices. The majority of those who had cervical cancer had used the Pill for more than 6 years. The other research group said that women under the age of 25 who used combination-type pills with a high synthetic progesterone level for at least 5 years had a 4 times greater risk of developing breast cancer than other women. In short, the Pill may be quite risky.

E. Butterworth, Jr., M.D., and Kenneth D. Hatch, M.D., along with their associates at the University of Alabama, have demonstrated that very large supplements of folate (a B vitamin) arrest and even reverse cervical dysplasia in just three months' time. Women taking a placebo instead of folate did not receive the same benefits. (The dosage is many times greater than the RDA, and the treatment is considered experimental.)

It's unclear how folate prevents the progression of dysplasia to cancer. Normal cell division, however, requires folate, among other nutrients. Dr. Hatch speculates that if folate levels in cervical tissues are low, there may be an increased chance of a mistake in cell division.

Women taking oral contraceptives should be especially careful, since their folate levels are typically low.

Another study showed that women whose Pap tests come back with shaky results or with a definite verdict of cervical dysplasia tend to eat much less food rich in vitamin A (beta-carotene, in particular) and vitamin C.

Today synthetic forms of vitamin A called retinoids are being tested on women who are likely to develop cervical cancer. By applying a vaginal salve containing these retinoids, cervical dysplasia may be prevented from developing into cancer.

Women at risk for cervical cancer are those with a history of early sexual activity or many sex partners, the presence of herpes simplex Type II virus or papillomavirus (flat genital warts) and a habit of cigarette smoking. Women whose mothers took DES (diethylstilbestrol) during pregnancy are at risk of developing a rare form of cervical and vaginal cancer, and should be diligent about getting Pap smears and other special screenings recommended by their physicians.

While the cells of the cervix are readily available for examination, the cells of the ovary are not. And where uterine cancers "announce" themselves by abnormal bleeding and discharge, ovarian cancer is silent. Its symptoms (if they show at all) are obscure and may seem more like GI trouble: abdominal discomfort, abdominal distention, weight loss. By the time the cancer is large enough to be discovered, it is often advanced.

Pelvic exams sometimes detect cancer early, but surgery gives the final diagnosis. Here's what we know: Women from 40 to 60 account for 60 percent of all cases, with the risk increasing among women who are childless or postmenopausal, or who use ERT. The disease may "run in the family." Coffee drinking *may* be linked to it. And once again, high-fat diets are indicted as a possible cause.

STOMACH CANCER: DISEASE ON THE DECLINE

What's 5'8", weighs 200 pounds, is cold and impersonal and takes credit for a big drop in United States cancer rates?

If you're thinking it's an eminent doctor with a weight problem, guess again.

It's your refrigerator.

In the last 25 years, there has been a 60 percent decrease in stomach cancer. Refrigeration helps—a lot. Because cold allows foods to "keep" longer, cancer-causing preservatives need not be added. Likewise, meats don't have to be smoked to retard spoilage.

To help prevent stomach cancer, we can do the following things:

Avoid Foods Preserved with Nitrites and Nitrates. In the gastrointestinal tract, these chemicals interact with other substances, called amines, to form new, highly carcinogenic compounds called nitrosamines. Today, it's just as easy to buy foods without these preservatives. Read all labels carefully.

Avoid Salted, Smoked and Pickled Foods. They may also contribute to stomach cancer. In a country where preservatives and salted and pickled foods are a way of life, then, we would expect to see more stomach cancer. This is exactly the case in Japan, where the disease kills more people than any other cancer.

Endometrial: the dangerous presence of hypertension, diabetes and/or obesity; infertility; late menopause; and prolonged estrogen therapy. Cervical: early sexual activity; numerous sex partners; poor hygiene; use of birth control pills or the IUD; cervical dysplasia; and continued use of oral contraceptives after diagnosis. Also at risk are DES babies.

Don't Eat Grilled or Fried Foods Every Day. Cancer-causing substances in meat and fish can be produced by these cooking methods—even when no nitrites are added.

Barraging the stomach with these potentially dangerous foods is bad enough. But the danger can be compounded by a lack of certain vital vitamins and minerals.

Low levels of selenium are very strongly linked to stomach cancer. And low levels of vitamins A and E amplify the effects of that deficiency.

In addition, vitamin E directly blocks the formation of nitrosamines. Vitamin C does the same. Toronto scientist Elizabeth Bright-See, Ph.D., of the Ludwig Institute for Cancer Research, says, "While attempts are being made to eliminate nitrates from foods . . . the most effective approach is surely to block nitrosamine formation before it occurs. For this purpose, vitamin C and E are important reactants."

In countries where people eat lots of smoked or pickled foods, rates of stomach cancer are higher. Regard these food products as an occasional treat.

PROSTATE AND BLADDER CANCER

Why are blacks living in North America ten times more likely to get prostate cancer than blacks in South Africa? Doctors from the American Health Foundation say it may be due to their diet. South Africans eat a low-fat, largely vegetarian diet; Americans eat a diet high in fat, high in meat. Even within the United States, rates for prostate cancer are higher in areas where people traditionally eat greater amounts of fatty food. And when researchers put American men on a low-fat, vegetarian diet, they see changes in their hormone levels—positive changes, such as lowered testosterone. Elevated levels of this hormone have been found in cancerous prostates.

Zinc also affects hormone levels. A University of Edinburgh study showed that "hormonal changes

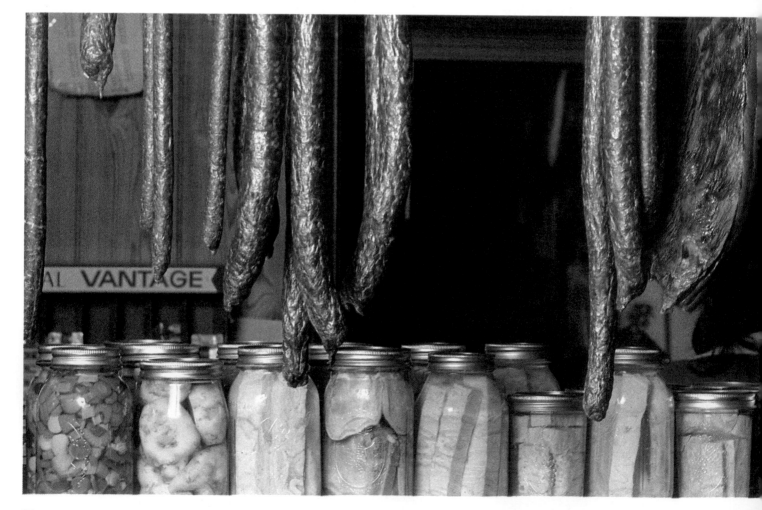

characteristic of the [prostatic] malignant tissue were only manifested after the zinc concentrations had reached . . . subnormal levels"— which implies a cancer-preventive role for zinc.

Signs of prostate trouble are urinary problems, back pain and painful ejaculation. Sometimes there are no symptoms, so regular rectal exams by a doctor are advisable.

"The incidence of bladder cancer is slowly rising, which may be due, in part, to the increasing use of chemicals in every phase of our modern society," wrote Mark S. Soloway, M.D., in the journal *Postgraduate Medicine.*

Among the chemicals implicated in this disease are those produced by smoking; trihalomethanes, which are found in chlorinated water; and artificial sweeteners.

Considering that 38,500 cases are diagnosed per year—and that many of those are already advanced

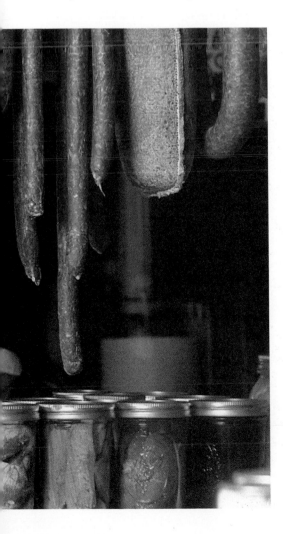

cancers—those risk factors are not to be taken lightly. Nor should symptoms of bladder cancer—bloody urine, too-frequent urination or difficult and painful voiding—be ignored.

Avoiding cigarettes and unsafe sweeteners and drinking bottled water are aggressive preventive steps. Ensuring that the diet is rich in vitamin A also helps. Important new research has shown that the bladder seems to be very sensitive to vitamin A levels, and that low levels were found in those suffering from bladder cancer.

IT'S UP TO US

We've seen that cancer is not really an amorphous enemy in our midst. This terrible disease is not inevitable; many types of cancer are, in fact, avoidable.

"Our knowledge of the causes of cancer is already sufficient to allow us to avoid more than half our present risk of cancer," says Dr. Arnold Reif. And, he predicts, "80 to 90 percent of the present incidence of cancer should eventually be preventable."

5

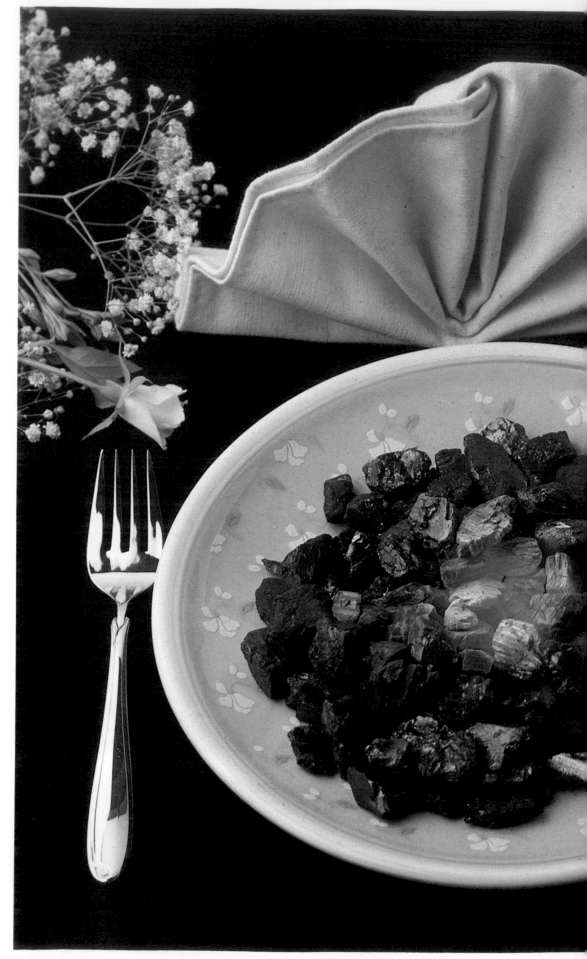

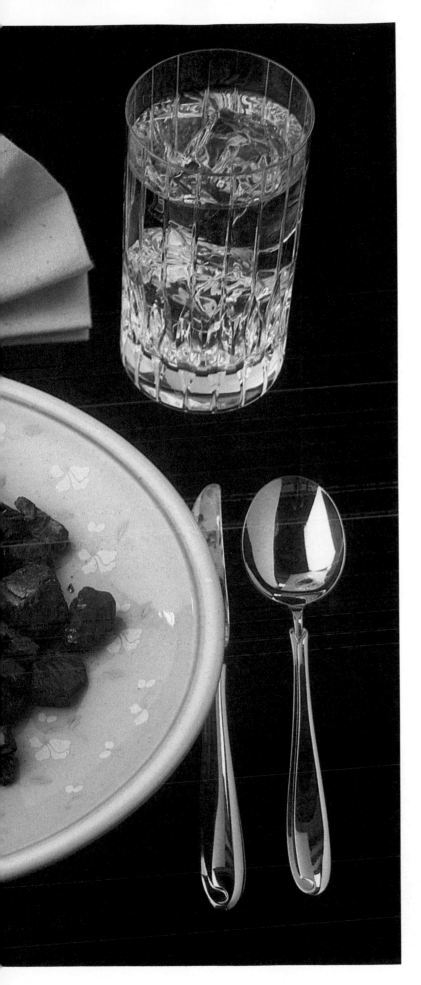

Upper Digestive Problems

Take the heat out of heartburn and ulcers. Using diet, combat gallstones and kidney stones.

This is a story of love—the *inside* story. Laurie is tired from hours of scanning figures in the office, and her mind is lost in thoughts of dinner with Jake. They are falling for each other and as Laurie waits for the elevator she gets a sudden craving for chocolate. She is not hungry, just tired and anticipatory. She knows, unconsciously, that the chocolate will soothe both feelings. It has always worked before. The bell rings and the elevator door opens to reveal a crowd. Laurie squeezes in and pulls a foil-wrapped package from her purse. The chocolate is from Switzerland, snugly contained, coddled in elegant European wrapping. Laurie tears the package open roughly. The chocolate melts in the heat from the crowd and Laurie unselfconsciously licks the smeared foil like a child as the elevator door opens. The chocolate is becoming part of her. Outside, the foil wrapper blows down the street as Laurie's molars reduce the chocolate to paste. Her tongue rises, squishing the sweet, brown candy against the roof of her mouth and then forcing it back into the contracting muscles of the throat and esophagus. The chocolate is squeezed along, like a rat being eaten by a snake, toward the pear-shaped sack of corrosive acid Laurie calls her stomach.

The lower esophageal sphincter opens, letting the chocolate into the pit. The expensive candy bar is just mush in the inferno, surrounded by tissue that is ridged like shallow canyons in an Arizona wash. The canyons contract, kneading the chocolate into a semiliquid mixture called chyme. Acid and enzymes break down the candy until, chocolate no longer, it is squeezed into the duodenum for the long trip through the body. The sugar has given Laurie a hard jolt of energy, and she feels warm as, at the restaurant, the maitre d' greets her. Jake is sitting at a corner table.

The upper digestive tract is a continuous

Bosses Give Ulcers, Not Get 'Em

It is time to give credit where credit is due. The bossed suffer more than the bosses. According to a government study, workers are *more* likely to experience stress-related illness, such as ulcers, than the big cheese upstairs.

The jobs associated with the most stress-related illness, ranked in descending order, are: laborer, secretary, inspector, lab technician, office manager and foreman.

On the other hand, doctors, executives, lawyers and company presidents—those who give the orders rather than take them—were not even ranked. That's executive privilege.

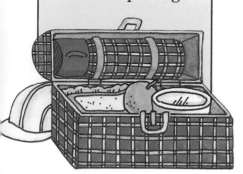

system. Laurie's started to work when she salivated at the first thought of eating the chocolate. Her saliva, esophagus and stomach worked together to prepare the chocolate so the intestine could absorb the nutrients. When the team is working well, the upper gastrointestinal (GI) tract is an efficient conveyer belt. But when something goes wrong with one part, the whole can be thrown off track. Fortunately, maintenance is not too difficult. With proper care— like good food and healthy habits— the upper GI will run smoothly throughout your life.

ULCERS: EXPLODING THE MYTHS

Ulcers were for a long time seen as a sign of success. Only someone with big pressures and a big ego got big ulcers. A hole in the stomach was as sure a symbol of lofty position as a silver Mercedes with a tinted glass sunroof. Well, ulcer's role as a status symbol has been debunked; the truth is that ulcers may occur more frequently in factory workers than in executives. And much of what scientists and doctors thought about ulcers—and how to cure them—has also been shown to be mythical. Fortunately, while the errors about ulcers were being revealed, other doctors were busy discovering natural treatments that actually work. But before we find out about them, let's look at just what an ulcer is.

Among ulcers of the upper digestive tract, the most common are duodenal and gastric, with the former occurring four times as frequently as the latter. Duodenal ulcers occur in the duodenum, located just below the stomach, where partially digested food first enters the intestines. Ulcers here tend to stage predictable, cyclical attacks during the day. They cause a gnawing, rhythmic pain in the upper middle abdomen that usually occurs a few hours after a meal. Some people are plagued by late-night pains that wake them up.

Gastric ulcers, however, are located in the stomach and give unpredictable, painful performances that may last for long periods of time. The pain is caused by self-cannibalization—the stomach eats itself. When everything is running smoothly, stomach acid and pepsin, an enzyme, break down the food in your stomach. Normally the lining of the stomach, called the mucosa, can withstand erosion by these digestive juices. But, for unknown reasons, the mucosa may weaken. Part may actually be digested, leaving an ulcer. Various factors, most of them controllable, can contribute to ulcer formation.

Occasionally an ulcer is so stubborn that it festers and recurs over a long period of time. Serious problems can then develop, including profuse bleeding and peritonitis (when the stomach contents spill through a hole into the surrounding tissue). These severe complications require emergency treatment, but they are uncommon and often preventable.

The first step to keep your stomach and duodenum happy is to watch what you put into your body. If possible, don't wait for an ulcer to occur and then try to cure it. Instead, prevent it from happening in the first place by treating your body well.

THE STOMACH AS AN ASHTRAY

Everyone knows that cigarettes cause major respiratory problems—the Marlboro man depends on his horse because he is too winded to walk— but many people don't realize that smoking also can contribute to ulcers.

According to Seymour M. Sabesin, M.D., professor of medicine at the University of Tennessee Center for Health Sciences, Memphis, there is sound evidence that associates smoking with ulcers. One possible explanation for the link is that smoking has been shown to interfere with the release of bicarbonate, a natural antacid, into the duodenum. And it doesn't help to switch to low-tar cigarettes; they're just as bad for you.

Do yourself a favor and kick the habit! (For specific details on how to calm a nicotine fit and succeed in quitting, see chapter 11.)

Aspirin, like cigarettes, can also

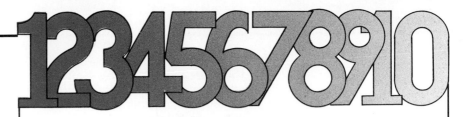

cause serious ulcer problems. It has been estimated that more blood is lost because of aspirin-induced stomach damage each year than is given in transfusions. The drug works directly on the stomach lining, irritating and sometimes ulcerating it. Medical studies have shown that people who take aspirin four or more days a week (or take 15 or more tablets a week) run a serious risk of suffering from acute gastrointestinal bleeding or gastric ulceration. It is clearly better to limit your aspirin intake whenever possible. (By the way, coated and buffered aspirins also damage the stomach lining.)

You might get a double dose of trouble if you use aspirin to soften the blow from too much alcohol. Two California doctors, Daniel Hollander, M.D., head of the division of gastroenterology at the University of California, Irvine, and Patsy Ann Hollander, Ph.D., a nutritionist in Newport Beach, warn that alcohol may be harmful because it stimulates stomach acid secretion. It has been established that alcoholics have more duodenal ulcers than nonalcoholics, and, according to Dr. Sabesin, excessive tippling may aggravate the symptoms of ulcers. It wouldn't hurt to drink fruit juice or mineral water instead of whiskey on the rocks next time the urge strikes.

STRESS AND ULCERS

Spirits of another kind also figure in ulcers. Anxiety and stress have long been thought to bring on ulcers. In fact, some people feel that the sharp rise in ulcers among women may be due to women taking more active—and stressful—positions in society. Ten years ago the incidence of duodenal ulcers in men was four to five times as great as among women; today almost as many women as men develop ulcers.

The link between stress and ulcers was even more graphically demonstrated during the prolonged bombing of London in World War II. Those who lived in the center of the city were hit regularly. They knew to expect fleets of bombers in the evening sky and lived their lives accordingly, always aware of where

Don't Blow Off Steam, Cool It Off Instead

If your ulcer acts up when the boss tells you to cancel your vacation because there are more important things to do, or your stomach gets tight when you hear the third baseball of the week smash through an upstairs window, you had better learn to control your anger. There is no way to halt the seemingly constant onslaught of life's little stabs. But there are ways to cool down under the collar when you feel someone breathing down your neck. The best way may *not* be the most common way—blowing your stack probably won't calm your body down. Maybe you should talk things out. Here are 5 tips from Solomon Schimmel, Ph.D., a psychologist from Brookline, Massachusetts:

Wait. Before you say or do anything . . . wait. Try anything (yes, even counting to 10) to give your anger a chance to pass or at least cool down. By delaying your response, you're less likely to do something you'll later regret.

Leave the Situation. If your anger is getting ready to boil over, try setting up a physical barrier (like leaving the room until you've cooled down), or a psychological barrier (like tuning out for a little while).

Interpret the Situation. Make yourself aware of the other person's behavior. Chances are you were wrong about their intentions. Once you realize they actually mean you no harm, you're less likely to explode.

Try to See the Lighter Side. Anger and humor are like oil and water; they just don't mix. If you look on the lighter side of a tense situation, you may succeed in getting everybody to laugh and cool down a bit.

Think about Anger. When you're in an anger-provoking situation and later, when you are not, think about what anger really is. It's a dangerous emotion that can be very harmful to you—and your ulcer. It accomplishes nothing. It makes you look foolish. It leads to things that you will regret later. Getting hold of your anger is worth the effort.

Doctors for years added punishment to pain when they ordered patients to control their ulcers by avoiding exciting, good-tasting, spicy foods. Bland, boring and basically "blah" foods like milk toast, cream of wheat, oatmeal, boiled eggs and saltines were thought to be easier for the sore stomach to handle.

Fortunately, ulcer-ridden gastronomes have been granted a reprieve. The Sippy ulcer diet (named for the man who promoted it) has been pulled from the menus of all but the most behind-the-times hospitals. Doctors now realize that very few foods cause ulcer problems. Milk, surprisingly, is among the foods that do. Doctors now believe that this cornerstone of the Sippy diet actually may aggravate ulcers.

the nearest bomb shelter was. Their extreme stress was at least partially controllable. But for those on the outskirts of London, where the raids were much less predictable, the stress was greater. Brief lulls, where life seemed almost normal, were suddenly interrupted by savage bombing raids. These people experienced a 300 percent rise in the incidence of ulcers, while the rate in central London rose by only 50 percent. This suggests that gastric health can be improved if some care is taken to maintain control of one's life.

Israel Posner, Ph.D., suggests that "periods of psychological safety seem to insulate subjects from the harmful effects of stress." So, insulate yourself once in a while by going for a walk, exercising, taking in a movie or having dinner with friends. You *can* reduce the stress in your life by taking the time to relax. Few things in day-to-day life are worth suffering over.

Finally, there is a factor that contributes to ulcers that is

uncontrollable. Some people are destined to inherit a weakness toward developing them. Studies show that people whose parents have had ulcers are three times as likely as others to be afflicted. But just because you are genetically marked doesn't mean you have to suffer.

You can prevent ulcers even when faced with high levels of stress or a hereditary risk. Diet is the key. And even if you already suffer from ulcers, there are several safe, natural ways to heal them and keep them from recurring.

One remedy being looked at now seems too easy and too cheap to be true. But it also seems to work. The cure is ordinary water.

DISCOVERING THE WATER CURE

It is 1980 in Tehran, Iran. The American hostages are the subject of mass demonstrations, Ronald Reagan and Jimmy Carter are facing off in a final showdown and America doesn't know what to make of the Ayatollah.

One victim of the revolution is F. Batmanghelidj, M.D., who is serving time in Tehran's Evin prison, "waiting clarification" of his "situation." Many of the prisoners in Evin are held in a similar "situation." Uncertainties about their status combine with the physical hazards of confinement to induce extreme physical and mental stress. Dr. Batmanghelidj sees ulcer pain all around him, sometimes so severe that it limits the prisoners' precious, stress-relieving sleep. Antacids are available, but nothing seems to work for the inmates.

One gray evening, a prisoner writhes on his cot in pain, clutching his stomach and thinking about the various treatments that have failed him. An ulcer that had been previously diagnosed by X ray has returned once again and he can find no relief.

He approaches Dr. Batmanghelidj, who, out of desperation, tells him to drink two glasses of water. The prisoner does so and, as the minutes pass, so does his pain. In the time it takes to get ready for sleep, the pain is gone.

Dr. Batmanghelidj is out of prison now and continues to look into

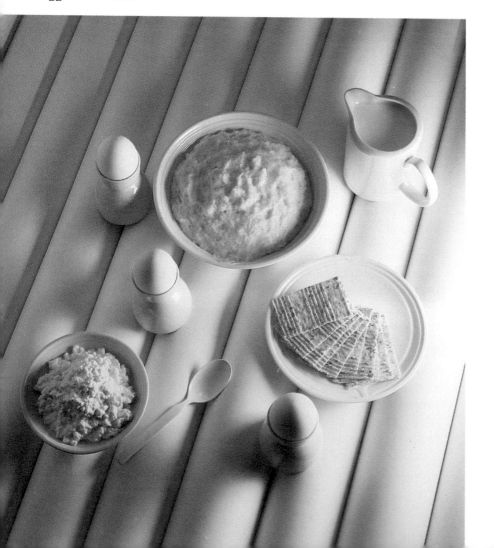

the water therapy. He saw more than 3,000 people with ulcers during the 2½ years he was imprisoned, and he came up with the following therapy. Drink one glass of water half an hour before each meal and another 2½ hours after each meal, for a total of six glasses a day. Continue the treatment for four to six weeks. The doctor is not certain why the therapy seems to work, but he believes that the "proof" surrounding the effectiveness of certain ulcer drugs may be due to the water used to wash down the numerous pills. While this treatment has not been clinically proven, water certainly won't hurt you. And it might be just what you need.

THE CABBAGE TREATMENT: A DOCTOR USES HIS HEADS

Another unusual treatment—this one *has* been proven—is found in cabbage leaves. The juice of the leaves, which can be extracted with an electric vegetable juicer, has been used to treat ulcers since the 1940s, when Garnett Cheney, M.D., fed ulcer patients 4 to 5 ounces of cabbage juice and 1 to 2 ounces of celery juice five times daily. Almost 85 percent of the subjects' ulcers healed within six to nine days. Seven years later, Dr. Cheney healed over 90 percent of a group of ulcer patients with cabbage juice concentrate. Nothing much was done with the research—there isn't much money to be made in cabbage juice futures—until Hungarian scientists found in the 1960s that a "great majority" of 162 ulcer sufferers received "complete relief from pain" after undergoing therapy with a derivative of cabbage juice. The juice can be made more palatable by adding other fresh vegetable juices such as celery and tomato. Drink it cold and toast your health.

The substance in cabbage that heals ulcers has not been isolated, but it may be a vitamin. Certain ones have been shown to help ulcer patients. Vitamin A, for instance, may do quite a bit more than help people see better on moonless nights; it has been used effectively to help prevent and even heal ulcers caused by extreme physical stress. Burn victims commonly suffer serious ulcers. In one study, 15 out of 22 burn or accident victims given the usual treatment and hospital nutrients developed stress ulcers. But in another group that was given vitamin A, only 2 out of 14 developed ulcers.

The vitamin may also help prevent gastric ulcers from turning into gastric cancer—a rare but frightening proposition. So, eat like a rabbit. High levels of vitamin A are found in spinach and other dark green, leafy vegetables, and in yellow and orange vegetables like carrots, pumpkins and squash.

You can boost vitamin A's effects with zinc, because zinc helps the liver distribute vitamin A in the body. The mineral has also been shown to help heal various types of ulcers, including stress ulcers in the stomach. Though it is a mineral, zinc is found in places other than caves and mines. Nuts, wheat germ, cheese, eggs, lima beans and meat all have large amounts of zinc.

Don't stop with vitamin A and zinc, however. One study—this involving laboratory animals—showed that vitamin E can help prevent stress ulcers from developing in the first place. To achieve this protection from vitamin E, eat peanuts, almonds and wheat germ with your vegetables.

When eating these and any other foods, it is a good idea to chew them well. The digestive process starts in your mouth, and the less work that has to be done in the stomach, the better. When you chew, you also mix in urogastrone, a substance in saliva that protects the lining of the duodenum from erosion. Chewing thoroughly also can help you lose weight by slowing down the pace of eating. It has long been known that the slower a person eats, the more satisfied he feels with less food.

Another way to get full and stay satisfied without overeating—and to prevent ulcers at the same time—is to eat large amounts of good-tasting, high-fiber foods. Fiber keeps the liquid part of a meal in the stomach longer. This mechanism appears to be protective, especially since we know that people with ulcers do not retain that liquid as long as healthy people.

The Ancient Drug-Free Ulcer Cure

Acupuncture, the ancient Chinese "needle" medicine, seems more like a torture than a cure to many Westerners. But is it really stranger than letting a doctor look into your stomach with a miniature camera? One study found that 63 percent of a group of 71 people recovered from their ulcers after acupuncture therapy. The ancient art offers healing without surgery, drugs or side effects—a good goal for Western medicine!

73

Doctors in Norway studied the effects of fiber on ulcers and came to the encouraging conclusion that a diet rich in fiber may protect against recurrent duodenal ulcers. The doctors had 38 people with healed ulcers increase their fiber intake by eating more whole wheat bread and whole grain porridge. Thirty-five other patients with healed ulcers were put on a diet low in fiber. The results were startling. Fully 80 percent of those on the low-fiber diet had another ulcer within six months. But only 45 percent of those on the high-fiber diet had any further problems during the study. Clearly, fiber can help you prevent ulcers.

Finally, a little romance may work wonders in combination with the above tips. Though some couples might find this hard to believe, connubial bliss has been shown to reduce the risk of ulcers in men. Maybe tying the marital knot lets the one in your stomach relax.

How Aspirin Ulcerates the Esophagus

Aspirin isn't always a pain reliever. For people who have hiatal hernias, it can be a pain inducer. The most common way hiatal hernias can irritate the body is by allowing stomach acids to backwash into the tender esophagus, causing pain and inflammation. But the inflammation can occur even without the acids.

In some people with hiatal hernias, an aspirin tablet won't move directly to the stomach, but will remain at the bottom of the esophagus. As it slowly dissolves there, it acts directly on the unprotected flesh, irritating it and possibly causing ulcers. When stomach acids have already damaged the tissue, aspirin makes for double trouble. The damaged tissue is more susceptible to the corrosive effects of aspirin than ever before. If you experience severe heartburn from esophagitis when you take aspirin, your cure for pain may be the culprit and halting your aspirin intake may solve the whole problem. Or, you might want to try an aspirin substitute to ease your pain. There is no reason to suffer more than you already do.

HEARTBURN: DON'T LIGHT THE FIRE

"I went to the club at lunch today. Aren't you proud that I'm doing the exercise you always say is so good for me?" says Jake, lighting a cigarette. "And I played Stanley a game of racquetball. He was fast—doesn't smoke—and whipped me right up and down that room. Couldn't do it in the boardroom, but on the racquetball court he has an advantage . . . anyway, the workout felt good."

"What did the scales say when you weighed yourself?" asks Laurie.

"Ah, c'mon. Let's just enjoy dinner. You know what they gave me for lunch after the workout? Health food! Some kind of Arab or African wood pulp all mixed in with tomatoes, peppers and some sort of flaked green things."

"Mint leaves, Jake. It must have been tabbouleh. I read somewhere it has fiber. Supposed to be food for . . ."

"So, I grabbed a pastrami sandwich on the way back to the office. Could you bring me another Scotch?" says Jake, lifting his glass toward the waiter.

"Have you lost any weight since you started?" quizzes Laurie.

"Well, two pounds this morning. But that could be because I skipped breakfast and weighed myself before lunch," Jake replies sheepishly. "Look, I know I've got to lose weight. But I can't eat any Middle Eastern wood pulp and still keep my strength up. And I've had such a burning pain in my chest that sometimes it's all I can do to make it through the day," he whines, taking a deep puff of his cigarette and exhaling a gray, lifeless cloud, which hangs above Laurie's head.

"Eat better, sweetheart," says Laurie. "You'll feel better."

It sounds like Jake is heading for trouble. Like so many of us, Jake makes big promises to himself that he doesn't keep. He is trying to exercise, but can't do very well because he smokes. He is trying to lose weight, he says, but isn't succeeding because he loves Scotch but hates "wood-pulpy" things like tabbouleh. The pain in his chest

Anatomy of a Hiatal Hernia

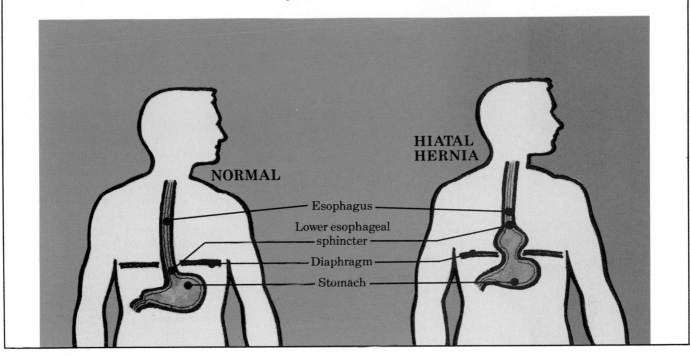

sounds like heartburn and, since he is overweight, chances are the heartburn is directly related to a hiatal hernia. Too bad. He possibly could have prevented his hiatal hernia without much trouble. Now that he has one, it will probably remain with him for life. But it needn't be the near-constant bother it is now. Jake can minimize the discomfort by cutting out a few things, such as alcohol and caffeine, and instead centering his diet on nutritious dishes that contain lots of fiber. It is simple. But you have to know how.

Hiatal hernias, like many digestive diseases, are common among Westernized people but very rare in traditional cultures. At least 20 percent of adults in the United States have a hiatal hernia. If you are 40 or older, according to some doctors, there is an even chance that you have one. Not everyone afflicted is aware of the problem; many hiatal hernias are unaccompanied by symptoms and cause absolutely no pain. So if a hiatal hernia shows up on an X ray but you don't feel anything, don't worry. Take good care of yourself (we'll show you how shortly), and you'll probably never have any pain.

A hiatal hernia occurs when excess pressure forces a portion of the stomach into the chest cavity, so it resembles a party balloon that has

been twisted to look like the head and torso of a dachshund. However, unlike balloon animals, hiatal hernias aren't much fun. They often mimic much more serious conditions like heart disease or disorders of the gallbladder or pancreas. Some people in the past even became cardiac "cripples"; their movement was severely restricted by doctors who diagnosed the pain caused by a hernia as a heart problem, when it really was nothing life-threatening. The hiatal hernia itself is painless, but the symptoms occur when the altered position of the stomach allows digestive acids to wash into the esophagus.

Even though few cases of hiatal hernia are so severe that they require surgery, many doctors operate on patients in an attempt to relieve the symptoms. Common methods involve sewing the stomach back into its proper position. Another, still-experimental procedure involves putting a collar that looks like an ox-yoke on the upper part of the stomach to prevent it from moving. Besides the normal complications associated with major surgery and anesthesia, these operations can fail when the pressure causes the sutures to tear through the tissue anchoring the stomach in place—and pressure is what hiatal hernias are all about. They result from strain: the strain of

The gentleman at left has a normal esophagus leading through the lower esophageal sphincter and into the stomach. The man at right is suffering from a hiatal hernia. His stomach has been forced up through the diaphragm so that it balloons into the chest cavity, straining the lower esophageal sphincter. This condition usually results in acid backwash, or heartburn. But it's easily cured by natural treatments.

being pregnant, being too full or being too fat, coughing, vomiting or sudden physical exertion. And most of these strains are preventable.

RELIEVING THE PRESSURE

The first thing you should do is lose weight if you are carrying excess pounds around. Extra layers of useless fat can increase the pressure in the abdomen, which may help shove the stomach into places it shouldn't be.

Do you remember the warm bran muffins your mother used to make—or you wished she would make—for you on cold winter mornings? You would smother them with butter and they would warm you up for the day ahead. But somehow you graduated to a quick cup of coffee and a sweet, sticky cheese danish once you moved out on your own, and you don't really know why. Well, give it up. That sticky danish does little for you except make you fat. And it doesn't have much fiber, either. Go back to your mother's menu, and fill up on high-fiber foods like bran muffins.

Fiber helps the food you eat pass quickly and easily through your system. A diet rich in refined carbohydrates and low in fiber will result in hard stools that are difficult to pass. According to Denis P. Burkitt, M.D., of St. Thomas Hospital Medical School in London, unnaturally high abdominal pressure is needed to evacuate the firm stools that result from a low-fiber diet. And this straining during defecation can cause a hiatal hernia. But increased intake of bran and other fibers will make everything easier—and will keep your stomach from sliding into your chest cavity.

Some people find breakfast the best time for bran, eating a muffin or a small bowl of bran flakes. And *small* is another key. Eating big meals creates an internal pressure that pushes the stomach up through the diaphragm. However, eating small meals throughout the day helps take the pressure off.

Severe coughing also can lead to hernia problems. In fact, smokers run a higher risk of developing a

hiatal hernia because they often have a persistent hack.

The really terrible part of a hiatal hernia is the tendency of the sufferer to experience esophageal reflux—that's when harsh stomach acid floods the lower esophagus, the bottom of the tube that leads from the throat to the stomach. The stomach lining is well protected by mucus (this is what helps keep ulcers from forming), but the esophagus is not. When acid repeatedly burns the lining of the esophagus, severe pain can develop, making people believe they are having heart attacks and other problems. Actually, it is the problem of the acid digesting the esophagus as it would a piece of steak. The resulting inflammation is called esophagitis. If esophagitis sounds bad, that's because it is. But not all hiatal hernias lead to it. And, there are many drug-free ways to control the condition when it hits.

ESOPHAGITIS: HEARTBURN WITHOUT THE HERNIA

Esophagitis can occur even without a hiatal hernia. The usual symptoms are heartburn and chest pain. Left untreated, severe esophagitis can result in swallowing problems. The esophagus and the stomach are separated by a doorlike muscle called the lower esophageal sphincter, which opens and closes automatically, perhaps in response to pressure. Normally, the lower esophageal sphincter exerts more pressure than the stomach, keeping the door shut against the stomach's contents.

But several things can cause a drop in pressure that allows the lower esophageal sphincter to open like a floodgate, letting acid into the esophagus to cause problems.

Coffee (regular *and* decaffeinated), alcohol and chocolate all weaken or relax that critical esophagus muscle. Even good-tasting and (usually) good-for-you dill and peppermint cause a drop in sphincter pressure. And cigarette smoking decreases the pressure dramatically. If you have trouble with heartburn, you might want to avoid all of these. Some people also avoid foods that directly irritate their acid-inflamed esophagus.

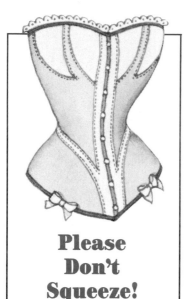

Please Don't Squeeze!

Though pinched waists, cummerbunds and broad, tight belts fade in and out of style, it might be best for the hiatal hernia sufferer to let others make the fashion statements. Tight clothes are out. Restrictive garments—even tight jeans—may actually make hiatal hernias worse. The hernias are caused by pressure. Don't increase it with form-fitting clothes. Stay loose!

These include coffee, tomato, spicy foods, alcohol and citrus fruit. Many people have found satisfactory alternatives to citrus fruit to meet their vitamin C needs, such as taking supplements or eating other, nonirritating foods that contain vitamin C, such as cabbage, broccoli and spinach.

Another common response to esophagitis is to down some antacids to neutralize those painful gastric juices. Yet medical studies have proven that these over-the-counter remedies are no more effective than placebos—compounds made of harmless, nonmedicinal ingredients. In fact, placebos may be *better* because many antacids contain aluminum, which interferes with the absorption of minerals important to healthy bones; calcium carbonate, which can actually *raise* the level of stomach acid; or sodium, which can contribute to high blood pressure.

Instead of antacids, try natural remedies such as dried grapefruit peel, papaya, parsley or celery. All these foods have worked for some people. Find those that work for you.

Here's another hint: To avoid symptoms while sleeping, raise the head of your bed on 6- to 8-inch blocks, so acid from your stomach won't be able to wash up into your esophagus. The law of gravity will keep the troublemaking liquid in your stomach. There is no need to be a victim of esophagitis. The natural cures are the cheapest, and they work the best.

GALLSTONES: EAT WELL AND AVOID THEM

The waiter, standing straight in a white shirt and black trousers, recites the menu in the hushed, serious tone that his customers expect. Jake is wealthy. He worked his way to the top and his preferred meals now are high-priced extensions of the un-healthy foods of his youth. He has traded the chicken-fried steak and country gravy of the past for expensive roasts and appetizers like butter-soaked escargot. The lamb arrives, glistening with fat that makes Jake drool. He punctuates a remark to Laurie by plopping a chunk of his

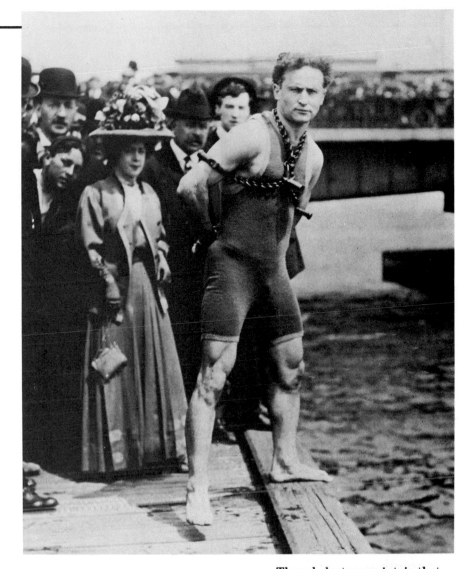

Though doctors maintain that the esophagus consists of involuntary muscle, carnival performers such as sword swallowers and escape artists have somehow learned to open the upper esophageal sphincter at will. In fact, Houdini's "magic" escapes were due to his ability to hide keys in his esophagus. He'd cough up the key and unlock himself without anyone knowing!

baked potato into his mouth. The mixture of lamb drippings, butter and sour cream satisfies something deep inside his soul and he sighs with pleasure. Laurie smiles as he tips back more wine.

Jake doesn't know it, but he's setting himself up for trouble down the line. The fat, cholesterol and alcohol in his diet may be causing his body to form gallstones. He won't know until he has a painful attack, and it is likely that he will suffer one unless he gets wise. Let's hope for his sake that he does. Gallstones are easily prevented with proper diet and exercise, and it's never too late to start. Those who already have the problem may reduce the risk of recurrent attacks.

Aside from its bad reputation, most people know little about the gallbladder. The words bile and gall have come to mean anger and brashness, and it seems that all the small, pear-shaped gallbladder does is cause trouble. In fact, the gallbladder works hard, storing and concentrating the bile we need for good digestion. Unfortunately, it often turns into an inflamed depository for gallstones. Many people have their gallbladders surgically removed when this happens, but the body usually continues to function as well as always. The bile flows directly from the liver into the intestine, bypassing its usual storage in the gallbladder. The pain and cost of surgery may not be worth it, however. About 10 percent of all patients still suffer abdominal pain, even without their gallbladders.

Why do some people have healthy gallbladders while others are cursed with recurrent attacks caused by gallstones? The answer is cholesterol. Many things contribute to the buildup of cholesterol in the bile, including obesity, eating a diet high in fat, sudden fasting, and drugs that contain female sex hormones.

The natural production of female hormones probably has an effect on the cholesterol level of bile, making the stones prevalent among people who are 3-f: fat, female and forty. The risk greatly increases during pregnancy. Birth control pills also roughly double a woman's chances of developing gallstones. And, ironically, both men and women increase their chances of getting gallstones if they take certain blood-cholesterol-lowering drugs like clofibrate.

Women can't do much about their natural tendency to develop gallstones, but they can forgo using birth control pills and take special care to avoid high-cholesterol foods. While everyone eats foods that contain varying amounts of cholesterol, some people go overboard, consuming lots of animal fats like well-marbled meat, butter and cream. As a result they acquire especially high levels of cholesterol in their bodies. When levels are too high, gallstones can develop. Here's how.

Surprisingly—and despite its bad press—cholesterol has a valid place in your body. It's found in some important hormones and in cell membranes. It is also the raw material from which bile acids are produced. These acids are extremely important to anyone concerned with gallstones. Found in the bile, they act like a detergent, breaking up the fat you've eaten. And if cholesterol is needed for the formation of bile acids, it should come as no surprise that it's also a constituent of bile. But your body needs only so much! When you eat foods containing a lot of cholesterol, the bile in your gallbladder becomes saturated with it, and the excess cholesterol starts to settle out. It forms crystals that clump together to become gallstones.

High-Fiber Recipe: Blueberry Corn Bread

Makes 10 servings

2 cups whole grain cornmeal
½ cup bran
1 teaspoon baking soda
1 teaspoon baking powder
1 cup blueberries
2 eggs
¼ cup maple syrup
1½ cups yogurt

Combine dry ingredients in a large mixing bowl; add blueberries and toss to coat. In a medium mixing bowl, beat eggs, adding maple syrup and yogurt. Add to dry ingredients, stirring just enough to combine; the mixture may be slightly lumpy. Place batter in a lightly greased 8 × 8-inch baking pan. Bake in a preheated 425°F oven for about 25 minutes, until golden brown.

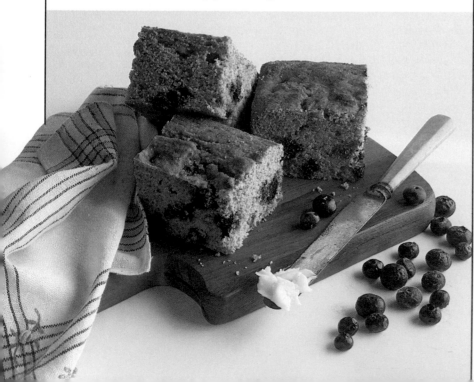

Most gallstones never cause a problem. They hide in the gallbladder or sneak through the body without ever causing pain. They can range from the size of a pinhead to almost as large as the gallbladder itself, and when they do flare up, they can cause extreme pain.

RESULTS OF OVERWEIGHT

One reason Americans suffer this pain so often is that many of us are overweight from eating a diet loaded with fat and sugar. Numerous studies have shown that obese people have bile that is packed with cholesterol—even more than people of normal weight who eat high-cholesterol diets. The famous Framingham Study of 5,000 Massachusetts residents, for instance, showed that being only 20 percent overweight doubles a person's chances of getting gallstones. But when obese people lose weight they also lose cholesterol. In fact, the lower your weight, the less cholesterol your body produces.

The paradox of obesity and gallstone formation is that high-calorie diets have been shown to increase cholesterol saturation of the bile, *and so have very low-calorie diets.* To understand how this mechanism works, imagine bile acids as little sponges that can absorb a certain amount of cholesterol. Obese people secrete so much cholesterol that the bile acids become saturated. When they go on a severe diet, the body produces a little less cholesterol and much less bile acid. So, there is less bile acid in proportion to the amount of cholesterol and the saturation level rises. That means you should lose weight sensibly. Most doctors advise against skipping meals, for instance. French physicians studied a group of 47 women with gallstones and a control group of women who had normal gallbladders. They found that many of the women with gallstones skipped breakfast altogether or had a significantly longer break between dinner and the following meal. When a person does not eat for long stretches of time, the gallbladder doesn't secrete very much bile, and yet the level of cholesterol

High-Fiber Disease Fighters

Food	Portion	Total Fiber (g.)
High-fiber and bran cereals	½ cup	up to 13.5*
Baked beans	½ cup	8.3
Apple	1 medium	7.9
Broccoli, cooked	1 medium stalk	7.4
Coconut	1 piece (2″ × 2″ × ½″)	6.1
Spinach, cooked	½ cup	5.7
Blackberries	½ cup	5.3
Almonds	¼ cup	5.1
Kidney beans	½ cup	4.5
Cabbage, shredded, boiled	½ cup	4.3
Peas, cooked	½ cup	4.2
White beans	½ cup	4.2
Banana	1 medium	4.0
Corn	½ cup	3.9
Potato	1 medium	3.9
Pear	1 medium	3.8
Lentils	½ cup	3.7
Lima beans, cooked	½ cup	3.5
Sweet potato	1 medium	3.5
Pinto beans	½ cup	3.1
Peanuts, chopped	¼ cup	2.9
Brown rice, raw	¼ cup	2.8
Cornflakes	1 cup	2.8
Orange	1 medium	2.6
Raisins	¼ cup	2.5
Brussels sprouts	4	2.4
Peanut butter	2 tbsp.	2.4
Whole wheat bread	1 slice	2.4
Apricots	3 medium	2.3
Carrot, raw	1 medium	2.3
Beets	½ cup	2.1
Peach	1 medium	2.1
Zucchini, raw	½ cup	2.0
String beans, raw	½ cup	1.9
Puffed wheat	1 cup	1.8
Tomato, raw	1 medium	1.8
Barley, raw	½ cup	1.6
Miller's bran	1 tbsp.	1.6
Onions, cooked	½ cup	1.6
Strawberries	½ cup	1.6
Walnuts, chopped	¼ cup	1.6
Asparagus, chopped	½ cup	1.2
Cherries	10	1.1
Cauliflower, raw	½ cup	1.0
Pineapple	1 slice. (3½″ diam. × ¾″ thick)	1.0

*Cereals vary in fiber content. Check individual product for specific information.

Surgery— No Cure for Gallstones

It isn't always wise to agree when your doctor says, "It's time to take out that gallbladder." Many gallstones never cause pain. Chances are only about 1 in 3 that these "silent" gallstones will ever require surgery. If you are over 60 years old, it might be best to avoid surgery altogether, because the risks on the operating table are too great. And even after surgery, 1 of 10 people still suffer some of their old symptoms. So, surgery should be thought of as a last resort except for severe gallbladder symptoms that might make a meeting with the scalpel unavoidable. Try the alternatives first.

secretion stays the same. What results is supersaturated bile. It might be wise to eat smaller, frequent meals, or at least eat breakfast every day in order to balance the cholesterol and bile acids in your system. Crash diets put a strain on the body and may even lead to developing gallstones.

Once the pounds are off, the amount of bile acids you produce will stabilize and the cholesterol saturation will be normal—not exaggerated as it is in obese people.

Exercise is important if you want to slim down. Swimming and walking are ideal exercises for the overweight. Or, try tennis or jogging if you aren't too heavy. Start off slowly and build up your endurance. Learning to exercise, like learning anything else, takes time and effort but pays off in the end. Any exercise you do will help. Not only will you lose extra pounds, but you may also lose extra cholesterol. It seems that exercise lowers the amount of cholesterol in the bile, reducing your chances of getting gallstones.

Another step to help you lose weight and fight gallstones is to eat a diet high in fiber. Some people—like Jake—think of sawdust in a pile under a carpenter's workbench when they hear the word fiber. But many delicious, filling, low-calorie foods are high in fiber. Chances are that some of them are long-time favorites— potatoes, fruit, berries and more. Studies have shown that fiber may play a great part in preventing gallstones from forming. Two Canadian physicians told the Royal College of Physicians and Surgeons of Canada that a diet high in refined carbohydrates increases bile cholesterol, while a diet rich in wheat bran fiber greatly reduces bile cholesterol levels. Societies that depend on fast food (high in refined carbohydrates, low in fiber), may encourage gallstone formation. Australian researchers also showed that a diet rich in wheat bran fiber may help prevent gallstones, and suggested that coarse bran flakes may work better than fine bran.

Vegetable fiber also plays a role. Researchers in Italy studied gallstone formation in 320 people and what they found confirms the benefi-

cial aspects of dietary fiber and the harmful effects of refined sugars. Half of the subjects suffered from gallstones and half were free of gallstones. The physicians analyzed the diet of the patients over a five-year period and found that the gallstone patients ate less vegetable and fruit fiber and more refined sugar than the healthy patients. The conclusion seems clear: Eat more fiber.

In addition, it may help to supplement your diet with vitamin C and zinc. Vitamin C has been shown to increase the rate at which cholesterol is changed to bile acids in test animals. There is good reason to believe that the same thing occurs in humans. Another study involving laboratory animals, with great potential effect for man, was done on the effects of zinc on gallstone formation. William H. Strain, Ph.D., and his colleagues in the department of surgery, Cleveland Metropolitan General Hospital, wrote that "zinc deficiency may be a factor in the development of gallbladder disease," and that "increased dietary zinc intake may help prevent gallstone formation and gallbladder disease." They seemed convinced that the findings from the studies done on animals are pertinent to humans, and urged further investigation. But there is no reason to wait passively for the results. Increase the zinc in your diet by eating more liver, cheese, fish, nuts and whole grains.

So, the overall strategy for fighting gallstones is really quite simple: Lose weight, exercise, avoid high-cholesterol foods, watch your vitamins and minerals and fill your plate with high-fiber foods.

HELP FOR KIDNEYS THAT FORM STONES

Laurie gulps the water from her crystal glass, and asks the busboy for a refill. She picks at her poached salmon—she rarely eats meat—and grows anxious for more water. The busboy arrives and Jake smiles as she drinks from the glass.

Laurie's meal will work wonders for preventing a variety of diseases and, specifically, the disease of affluence, kidney stones.

Prevention, as usual, is much easier than a cure. All that's required are changes in diet and liquid intake. And these changes are well worth the effort, because once a stone is lodged in the kidney, nothing short of surgery—which can result in the loss of part or all of the kidney itself—will get rid of it. So, avoid trouble in the first place by depriving your kidneys of the elements needed to form stones.

Kidneys regulate the body's fluids, which contain various minerals and other substances. Usually these flow out of the body if they are not needed. Trouble starts when there is too much of these substances and not enough fluid. The most common stones occur when calcium, a mineral, combines with a substance called oxalate in such great quantities that it cannot remain in solution. One small crystal will form, then attract another and another until a sizable stone develops. Usually the jagged-edged stones then pass through

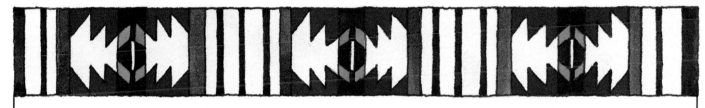

Pima Studies Show Cause of Gallstones

The Pima Indians are isolated from mainstream American culture in the hot Arizona desert south of Phoenix. Still, they have contributed more to scientific knowledge of gallbladder disease than any group in the world. The reason: Pima Indians have perhaps the highest incidence of gallstones of any population on earth. About 50 percent of the men and 70 percent of the women will develop gallstones by the time they are only 30 years old. This condition may be due to the obesity that resulted when the Pimas switched from a diet of whole grains and beans to one of refined carbohydrates and fats.

The Pimas lived healthy lives in the Gila River valley for 2,000 years, growing their own food on farms fed by highly advanced irrigation canals. The valley is one of the hottest and driest places on earth, but the Pimas were able to grow enough grain to feed many white settlers who moved to the area after the Civil War. The two cultures lived in relative harmony until the late 1800s, when the settlers diverted most of the river water, destroying the Pimas' agricultural base and making them dependent on Western ways—and food—to stay alive. The Pimas now consider obesity a sign of health, though 19th-century photographs show the Indians as being slimmer than they are today.

Each Pima has been offered a complete physical examination every 2 or 3 years since 1965 by researchers interested in collecting data on the various diseases that afflict the Indians. This research has led to the discovery of the connection between bile-cholesterol saturation, obesity and gallstones. Moreover, based on this and other data from this study, birth control pills now carry a warning about gallstone formation. It is hoped that the Pimas will continue to teach us how to control gallstones, while at the same time limiting their own health problem.

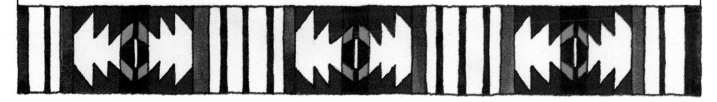

the urinary tract, searing the body with excruciating pain all the way. Sometimes, however, they get stuck and block the flow of urine. This condition requires surgery.

But standard medicine seems to be stabbing in the dark with the various less-than-successful treatments. According to a doctor at the University of Texas Health Science Center at Dallas, up to 70 percent of people treated with traditional methods can expect recurrences. You can prevent them by eating the right foods.

The stones are most prevalent in people who eat lots of meat and little fiber. Africans living in their tribal homelands who are not yet hooked on hot dogs, fatty foods and processed grains don't get kidney stones. The difference in the incidence of the disease is probably not racial—black Americans are susceptible to kidney stones, though not as susceptible as American whites. And in areas of South Africa where large groups of both whites and blacks eat a Western diet, the disease is rampant.

RICH FOODS, POOR HEALTH

Ernest Hemingway was correct when he wrote, "the very rich are different from you and me," not only because "they have more money," but also because they form more kidney stones. In this case, wealth is measured by the amount and kind of food available, and history shows that during times when food was scarce, so were kidney stones. The incidence of kidney stones in European countries during the world wars dropped significantly. Meat and dairy products were hard to come by due to the bombings and short-circuited supply routes. But when the fighting stopped, the diet "improved" and the incidence of kidney stones jumped. A later British study showed that the number of people with kidney stones fluctuated (with a two-year delay) between 1958 and 1976 in the same pattern that the amount of money spent on food did. More money spent equaled more kidney stones. Why? Because when people have the cash, they'll choose steak over beans and buy butter for their bread. Researchers have found a direct link between the amount of meat, fish and poultry a group of people eats and the number of kidney stones they'll get. Researchers in Vienna found that meat eaters excrete significantly higher levels of calcium than do people who prefer vegetables. Thus, more calcium passes through the kidneys, increasing the likelihood of stone formation.

Stop those stones before they stop you! Save money and your

A Cheap Cure for the Disease of the Rich

Long called "the disease of affluence" because it goes hand in hand with a rich diet, recurrent kidney stone disease may respond to an inexpensive cure. Water will flush the kidneys clean. "It is the best and safest treatment for most patients with kidney stones," says William D. Kaehny, M.D., of the University of Colorado. He recommends downing 16 glasses of water a day and setting an alarm clock to wake you in the middle of the night so you can pass the water and drink more. Most people, says Dr. Kaehny, won't develop a second stone if they put themselves on the water therapy.

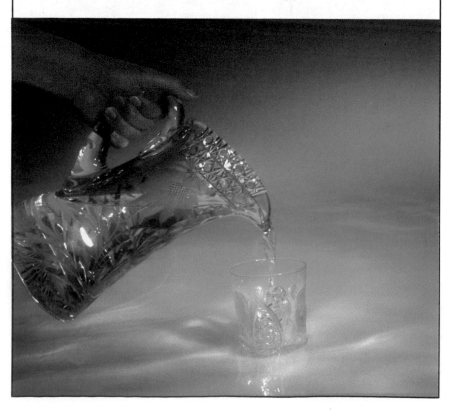

kidneys at the same time by cutting down your intake of animal protein.

At the same time, eat more whole grains, vegetables and fruits, all of which are high in fiber. Sugar and other refined carbohydrates such as white flour and rice—all common in affluent societies—may encourage the formation of kidney stones by increasing the amount of calcium in the urine. British researchers found a direct link between kidney stones and a diet high in sugars. Eighteen patients were tested for urinary calcium while alternately eating diets with low, normal and high amounts of sugar. They showed sharp increases in urinary calcium while on the high-sugar diet. But fiber found in wheat bran and brown rice may prevent kidney stones from forming by lowering urinary calcium. A survey conducted in Ireland showed that people with kidney stones ate less fiber than those without stones. But don't use fiber as an antidote for bad foods. Let it replace them.

While you are improving your diet with fiber, also evaluate the nutrients in the food you eat. Consider taking supplements of vitamin B6 and magnesium. They help prevent kidney stones from forming. People often criticize others who take supplements, saying that the vitamins and minerals just leave the body, giving "health nuts" the most expensive urine in town. While it is true that many nutrients are excreted, they are not necessarily wasted. Alan Gaby, M.D., a family practitioner from Baltimore, Maryland, says that these "wasted" vitamins may promote good health in the kidneys by their presence in the urine. According to Dr. Gaby, a large amount of "wasted" magnesium in the urine actually reduces the risk of calcium stone formation. Like calcium, magnesium, which has been used to treat kidney stones since 1697, can bind with oxalate in the urine. When calcium and oxalate bind, they often form stones, but magnesium is less likely to form stones when it meets oxalate. With magnesium and calcium competing for the oxalate like two bidders at an auction trying to buy the same Tiffany lamp, the chances of calcium winning are reduced—along with your chances of

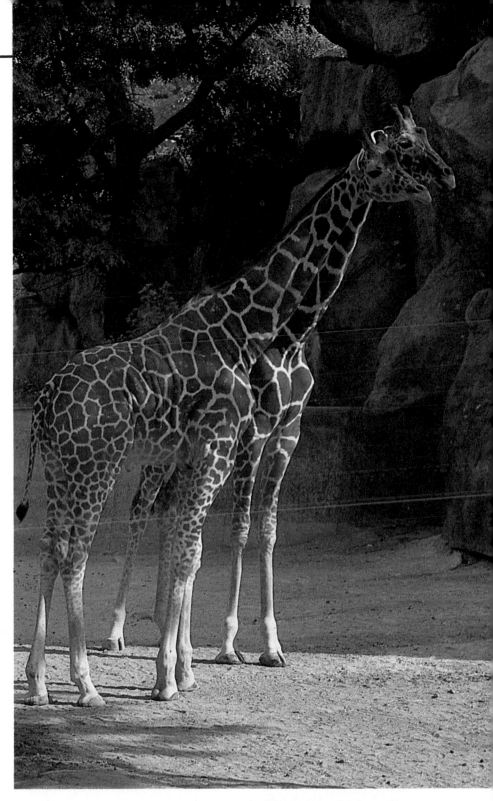

getting a kidney stone.

Swedish researchers tested this theory by giving 200 milligrams of magnesium per day to 55 people who averaged about one stone per year. After two to four years of therapy, only 8 of the patients formed new stones. As a group, their average rate of developing new stones fell by 90 percent, compared with a recurrence rate of 59 percent in a group who didn't take magnesium. Magnesium

This isn't a tall tale at all, but it might be hard to swallow. Even giraffes get kidney stones. An animal physiologist from Kenya studied 75 giraffes in South Africa and found that 22 of them had kidney stones.

Vitamin E for Jaundice Puts Babies in the Pink

Doctors in 1958 discovered that babies who spent their first days on the sunny side of nurseries didn't exhibit any signs of the common liver ailment, jaundice. Long-term doses of artificial light— phototherapy— became standard jaundice treatment at hospitals. Researchers now know that such long-term treatment may cause genetic damage, but vitamin E has come to the rescue. A study showed that premature infants who are given vitamin E in their first few days of life have less of the jaundice-causing substance in their blood than babies who don't get the vitamin. They also don't need to spend as much time under artificial light to get rid of the sickly yellow color that goes along with jaundice, thus minimizing the sick infants' chances of developing genetic problems.

is found in green, leafy vegetables, and in nuts, peas, brown rice, soybeans and whole grains.

And, researchers in Boston conducted a long-term study of 149 patients that showed a 90 percent cut in calcium oxalate stone formation after daily nutritional therapy. The nutrients: magnesium and vitamin B_6. The latter vitamin, found in bananas, whole grains, salmon, filberts, poultry and tomatoes, has been proven to be an effective oxalate fighter. Researchers in India discovered that 10 milligrams a day of vitamin B_6 "significantly" lowered the amount of urinary oxalate in people prone to forming kidney stones. They found that B_6 worked more efficiently than thiazides. These are diuretics commonly used to treat high blood pressure, but they are also used to prevent kidney stones by increasing the urinary output. That is good news, because thiazides also can cause light-headedness, promote diabetes and gout and reduce the amount of potassium in the blood, causing muscle weakness and cramps.

Vitamin B_6 got another boost when researchers reported that a woman who was passing stones daily found great relief with the vitamin. She had suffered from recurrent stones for 20 years, but after she was given high doses of B_6, the woman's urinary oxalate dropped to the normal range. She continued taking B_6 and her condition remained stable. Combine vitamin B_6 and magnesium with a low-meat, low-fat diet full of fiber and lots of fluids, and you will probably never need to try Ben Franklin's "cure." He stood on his head and ate blackberry jelly in an attempt to dislodge a kidney stone.

THE ESSENTIAL LIVER

"Oh, my!" Laurie exclaims to Jake as the flames flicker to oblivion, leaving a chafing dish of slightly warmed pears in brandy.

Jake forgoes the sweets, and instead orders his brandy straight. "Watching the weight, you know," he slurs. The waiter brings the delicate balloon-shaped glass. Laurie refrains from commenting on Jake's alcohol consumption as he sips the potent liquor. Laurie knows he is changing his habits for the better, though ever so slowly. She thinks he had better hurry, though, before his liver gives out.

Alcohol is used to seal agreements, to celebrate unions and to commemorate the happy occasions in life. Unfortunately, alcohol is frequently abused to the point of causing one of the most debilitating and frightening (because it can't be reversed) diseases that afflicts modern man: alcoholic cirrhosis.

The liver is the sewage treatment plant for the body. It filters the blood, processing nutrients from digestion while also detoxifying drugs and other foreign substances. That's how the liver works when it's working well. But this sensitive organ is easily damaged by onslaughts of alcohol, which is broken down by the liver. In the process, the liver itself can be broken down. A cirrhotic liver is actually a scarred liver, one so badly injured that it can't be restored. Alcohol is the primary cause of such damage and although other, non-alcohol-related problems may lead to the disease, cirrhosis is more common in alcoholics than it is in nondrinkers.

It normally takes a long time for the alcoholic to develop cirrhosis— the first stages are usually a fatty, swollen liver and alcoholic hepatitis, both of which may subside when the person ceases to drink. But once cirrhosis sets in, it can't be reversed.

Despite this, someone who has developed cirrhosis shouldn't give up hope and continue to drink his life away, because the liver can continue to function—though not at optimal level—if the person stops pouring glasses of wine or double martinis down the hatch.

That step is not always easy, though. Alcoholism is a serious disease in itself, aside from cirrhosis, and cures are very difficult. Consultation with a doctor, psychologist or a self-help group for alcoholics is a good way to start to look for help. (For good tips on quitting alcohol, see chapter 11.)

Besides going on the wagon, the best way to fight the ravages of cirrhosis is through diet. Eating properly prevents the occurrence of other diseases like severe dermatitis from a lack of zinc, night blindness from a deficiency of vitamin A, mental dysfunction from too few B vitamins and a host of other problems, including scurvy, that can go hand in hand with cirrhosis.

Once alcohol intake has been controlled, your body should be treated to a different sort of cocktail. Try fresh fruit juices to restore the body's levels of vitamins. Mixing fresh orange juice in a blender with a small amount of brewer's yeast is a good way to enjoy a cool drink and build up the body's supply of the B vitamins and vitamin C. And you won't regret it in the morning.

Vitamin A, commonly found in carrots, broccoli, liver and spinach, is very important to those fighting liver disease. It is directly related to night blindness—a common problem among cirrhotics because they suffer from vitamin A deficiencies. But just eating foods rich in vitamin A may not be enough.

Zinc has a curious way of boosting the effectiveness of vitamin A. It seems that the mineral is necessary to help the liver circulate vitamin A through the bloodstream. Alcoholics can be very low in zinc at the same time that they are low in vitamin A. But zinc does more than just help vitamin A circulate in your body. Lack of zinc causes acrodermatitis enteropathica, a serious skin disease that occurs in infants who, due to a hereditary disorder, are unable to metabolize this mineral properly. Impaired liver function in alcoholics can cause a zinc deficiency that mimics the symptoms of that disease. It causes inflamed and ulcerated skin, along with a loss of hair. But these symptoms can be avoided by eating the right foods. Zinc is found in large quantities in liver, meat, cheese, whole grains and nuts. One sign of a possible zinc deficiency is white spots on your fingernails. If you see these, you may need to add some of the above foods to your diet. While the cirrhotic liver will never return to its optimal state of health, a good, alcohol-free diet will do miraculous things for the sick person's energy level, appearance and outlook.

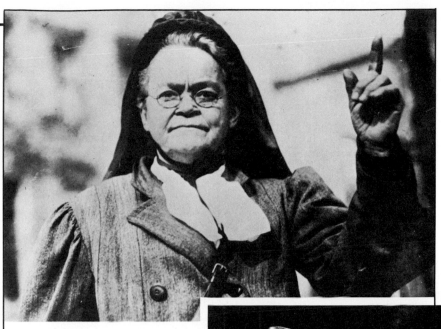

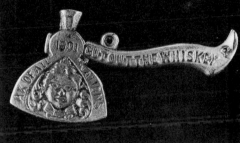

Dried-Out Country Dries Up Liver Disease

Carry Nation kept a lot of people healthy by seeing the devil in the bottle and leading the fight for forced temperance. When the Prohibition-era G-men broke down warehouse doors and smashed open giant wooden kegs of beer and whiskey, they were doing more than keeping people from weaving through the streets in intoxicated revelry; they were keeping the country safe for healthy livers. Cirrhosis took 11 in 100,000 lives before Prohibition, but the rate dropped to 7 in 100,000 during the period of forced abstinence. Repeal sent the rate right back up to the pre-Prohibition figure.

Jake winces as he signs the check, and both he and Laurie chuckle. Their time together has been worth the cost. Jake is a little bloated and foggy, but he suggests that they take a walk.

The traffic flows down the avenue in a great rush as they walk arm in arm. Jake pauses and prepares to light a cigarette, but changes his mind and tosses the pack victoriously into a trash bin. He's going to make it this time.

Step by step the couple strolls through the evening. There is hope around each corner.

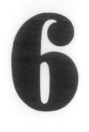

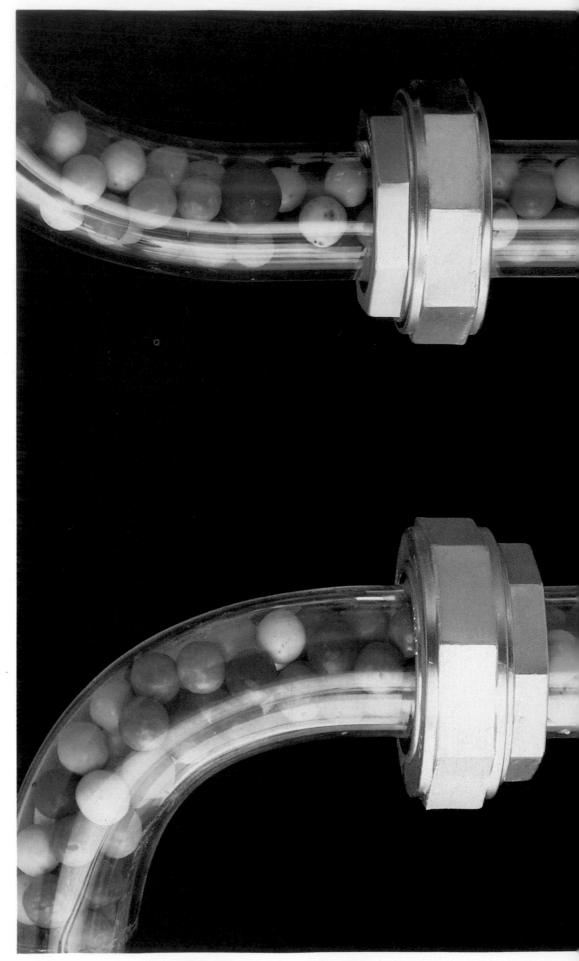

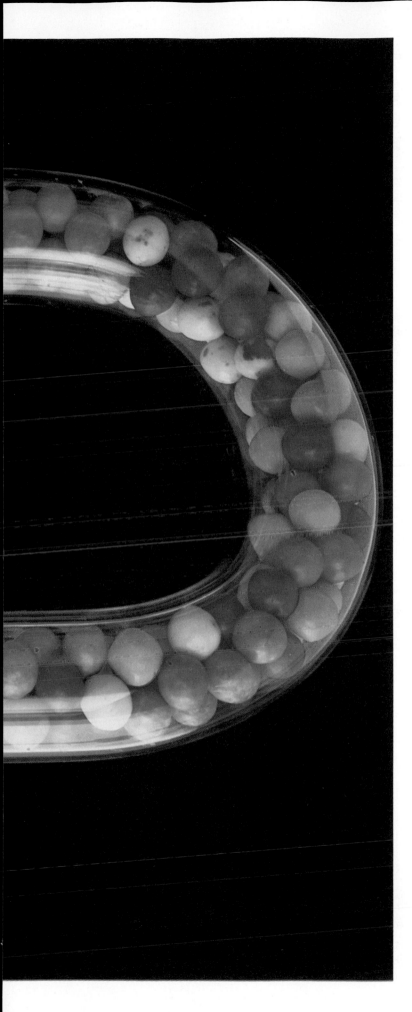

Calming a Stressed Intestine

Sorting the truth from the myths of digestive problems can spare you a lot of pain and indignity.

L ike a municipal waste disposal system, the lower gastrointestinal tract is designed to process the products of food digestion silently and efficiently. When it's in good working order, you're hardly aware of what's going on. But should something go wrong, the agony and embarrassment you suffer are unequaled.

Lower digestive tract ailments vary and include celiac disease, colitis, Crohn's disease, hemorrhoids, polyps and diverticulitis. This chapter also includes information about appendicitis and cystitis.

People with those diseases have much in common. Intuitively, they suspect that their troubles have something to do with food, so many experiment with their diet even before they seek medical advice. And, at some point, most wonder whether anxiety, depression or other emotional problems may be causing their condition.

Many lower digestive problems *do* stem from diet. But the issue of what you should or should not eat is a matter of much confusion and controversy. For years, doctors advised people with an irritable colon or diverticular disease to eat little or no roughage, otherwise known as fiber. Now, doctors realize that too little fiber *causes* those diseases.

Lactose intolerance, once regarded as a rare defect, is in fact more common than it is uncommon. Even appendicitis, which most people assume to be a completely unforeseeable emergency, might be forestalled by diet.

CELIAC DISEASE: LIFE WITHOUT WHEAT

If someone with celiac disease eats a slice of bread, the lower digestive tract goes into a rage, pumping out gas and copious, rank-smelling, frothy stool. If the disease persists, the person may begin to waste away.

How can all that turmoil result from eating a wholesome, innocent-looking slice of bread? For people with celiac disease, gluten—a protein in wheat—damages the intestinal lining, interfering with the way it absorbs nutrients from the food they eat.

Celiac disease seems to be an inherited tendency, although the exact cause is the Rubik's Cube of digestive puzzles—possibly a complex interlocking set of genetic factors, immune reactions and food chemistry. Thankfully, celiac disease is not only rare, affecting as few as 1 in every 1,200 people in this country, according to some estimates, but it

also is manageable. Obviously, it's most important to steer clear of foods made from wheat. You may be able to eat small quantities of other grains that contain lesser amounts of gluten—rye, barley, oats, malt and triticale. Tolerance varies from person to person; some people simply need to reduce their intake of gluten, while others need to eliminate it altogether. For those, the trouble-free grains are corn, rice and buckwheat.

Your first instinct—a correct one—will be to cut out most cereals, noodles and baked goods. To successfully avoid *all* sources of gluten, also sharpen your label-reading skills. For example, the following commercially prepared foods may contain wheat or other sources of gluten: luncheon meat, weiners, meat loaf, sausage, meat or fish patties and gravies; canned or frozen foods with thickened sauces; cheese spreads with cereal fillers; eggs in cereal-thickened sauces; puddings or casseroles with crumbs; thickened soups; bouillon cubes; coffee substitutes made with grains; beer, ale, whiskey, vodka, gin; commercial salad dressings thickened with a grain; soy sauce, some baking powder, cane sugar, molasses, chocolate candy; and communion wafers.

Life without wheat doesn't have to be difficult or dull. Look for products made of the previously mentioned corn, rice and buckwheat, as well as sorghum, tapioca, arrowroot and potatoes. Flours made from those starches offer both variety and good nutrition. Other wheat-free items to help you plan versatile meals that the whole family can enjoy include flours made from ground soybeans and garbanzo beans; amaranth flour; rice cakes and cereals; pasta made from corn, buckwheat, rice, arrowroot, mung beans or Jerusalem artichokes; wheat-free soy sauce or tamari sauce.

MAKING UP
FOR WHAT'S LOST

Because their intestines are in such an uproar, people with celiac disease frequently can't absorb all of the nutrients in their food. And they won't be completely well unless they

Once Again, Breast Is Best

Breastfeeding can prevent celiac disease in children otherwise destined to inherit the problem. Over the past few years, doctors have noticed that as more mothers breastfeed their babies, fewer children develop celiac disease. The doctors feel that the protein in cow's milk triggers gluten intolerance by damaging the intestinal lining, which in turn blocks the absorption of gluten, making it difficult to digest wheat and other grains.

The longer an infant is breastfed (and thus protected from gluten), the less likely the child is to develop celiac disease. Delaying the introduction of cereals to the diet for 4 to 6 months further helps to stave off celiac disease.

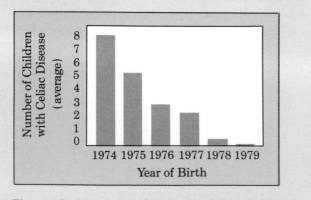

The graph above is based on the incidence of celiac disease observed in one clinic over a 6-year period.

take nutritional supplements to compensate for malabsorption. When supplementing, consider the following:

Zinc. Most of the zinc we get from food is thought to be absorbed in the duodenum and jejunum, which are the two intestinal areas hardest hit by celiac disease. Consequently, many people with this problem absorb little zinc from their food. That loss is all the more alarming when you consider that zinc is fundamental to healing.

Iron. While iron deficiency may take somewhat longer to show up than zinc deficiency, recovery will not be complete until iron is restored. In one study, British pediatricians discovered that of 91 children with celiac disease, 34 were anemic.

B Vitamins. At least one study has shown that many people with celiac disease frequently are low in folate, a B vitamin. Folate deficiency produces a number of distressing mental and physical symptoms, including diarrhea and cramping. Folate deficiency also can result in anemia—a common problem among those suffering from this disease, but perhaps even more common when folate levels are low. This anemia can lead, in turn, to fatigue and muscular weakness, adding to the misery of celiac disease.

Doctors have included celiac disease among the conditions that depress blood levels of vitamin B_6. And a shortage of this vitamin can contribute to the psychological depression so commonly suffered by people with celiac disease. Reporting this phenomenon in the *American Journal of Clinical Nutrition*, Swedish doctors recommended that vitamin B_6 supplements should always be added to a gluten-free diet for people with this problem.

Pediatricians in Finland studied vitamin B_{12} levels in 19 children with celiac disease. Their results indicated that many adults and older children with this problem run short of this vitamin. When the small intestine is damaged, diseased or surgically removed, B_{12} is not well absorbed. Unabsorbed, it is excreted.

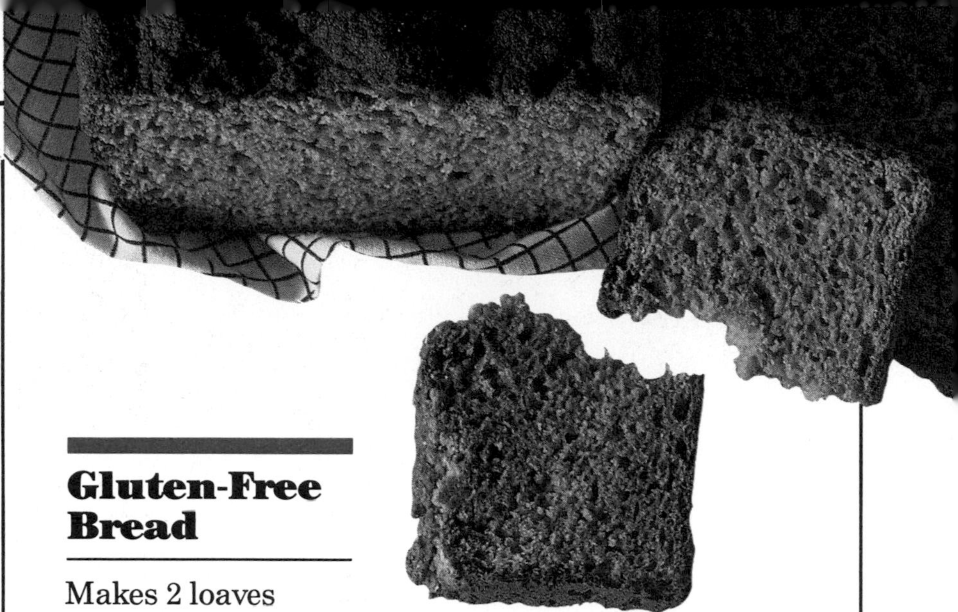

Gluten-Free Bread

Makes 2 loaves

1½ cups brown rice flour	4 egg yolks, beaten
½ cup soy flour	2 cups buttermilk
1½ cups rice bran	2 tablespoons oil
¼ cup potato flour	¼ cup honey
1 tablespoon baking powder	4 egg whites, stiffly beaten
1 teaspoon baking soda	½ cup raisins

Grease two 8 × 4-inch loaf pans. In a large bowl, sift dry ingredients together. Add egg yolks, buttermilk, oil and honey. Mix at low speed until well combined. Fold in egg whites and raisins last. Pour into prepared pans and bake in a preheated 350°F oven for 40 to 50 minutes.

You can compensate for this faulty absorption by saturating the system with those vitamins and minerals to ensure that *some* nutrients will reach their destination and thus prevent deficiencies.

A gluten-free diet, supplemented with vitamins and minerals, should put the digestive system back in working order. If this approach does not work, you may lack tolerance for other protein foods as well. One likely culprit is milk. In some people, intolerance to wheat can coexist with intolerance to lactose, the primary carbohydrate in milk. Therefore, begin by eliminating milk and all milk products, as well as all gluten, for a week, to see if symptoms ease. Occasionally, a person's intestines react poorly to proteins other than milk. If you suspect you have this problem, experiment by eliminating the most common sources of protein in your diet, one at a time: eggs for one week, then chicken, then fish, until you notice some improvement.

COLITIS: PUTTING A STOP TO "INTESTINAL HURRY"

Your stomach feels like it's clamped in a giant vise. You writhe in pain. When you go to the bathroom—which is embarrassingly often—you pass blood, pus and mucus with stools. Perhaps spending so much time in the bathroom makes you frequently late for work, annoying your boss. Shopping and car trips are risky because you never know where the nearest bathroom is. You fear that you'll soil your clothes. You also worry about that bleeding. Could it be cancer?

The cause of all that misery is ulcers in the mucous lining of your lower digestive tract, in the colon and rectum. Hence the name ulcerative colitis, or inflammatory bowel disease. Colitis can lead to polyps, hemorrhoids, abscesses, perforations—and possibly cancer.

A less serious type of colitis, called irritable colon and spastic or mucous colitis, is not as scary or as dangerous. Unlike ulcerative colitis, the intestines aren't inflamed, just irritated. Both types of colitis tend to strike without warning, making it difficult to lead a normal social or business life. Colitis of any kind can drain your energy, pummel your morale, put the kibosh on your sex life, and in general flush your self-image down the tubes.

But don't for one minute blame yourself for this disease—or blame the fact that you may deal poorly with stress. While stress may trigger flareups, the cause is not emotional in nature. Some doctors believe heredity may be a factor, others think the cause is a slowly developing virus. Most simply admit the cause is unknown.

If your doctor says you have "a touch of colitis," be sure to ask, "which kind?" The answer makes a difference in how to handle it. One of the biggest differences between spastic colitis and ulcerative colitis is the role of bran (or fiber, more accurately). For years, doctors recommended a bland, low-fiber diet for anyone with colitis of any sort. And that's certainly appropriate for people with ulcerative colitis. Fiber can lacerate an already ulcerated colon to the point where a person can bleed severely—and suffer unmercifully in the process. People with ulcerative colitis are better off avoiding raw vegetables, fruit and fruit juices when their colitis is bad.

For people with irritable colon, where no inflammation is present, doctors have found that fiber *can* help relieve constipation, diarrhea and abdominal cramps. Arthur D. Schwabe, M.D., professor of medicine and chief of gastroenterology at the University of California School of Medicine in Los Angeles, recommends a diet high in fruit and vegetables, plus 2 tablespoons of 100 percent whole bran a day. Frequent diarrhea can lead to dehydration very quickly. So be sure to drink six to eight glasses of water a day. And, along with one of those glasses, take a multiple vitamin and mineral supplement. Because some vitamins and minerals are normally absorbed in the portion of the intestinal tract where colitis occurs, people with this disease may not get all the nutrients they need. Moreover, bleeding drains the body of iron. The resulting subpar nutrition can account for the lack of energy common to colitis.

Ulcerative colitis tends to first appear in the twenties or thirties, but it may also first strike between age 60 and the late seventies.

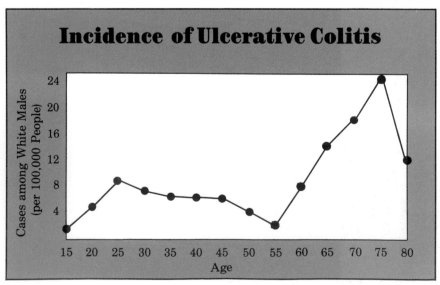

Incidence of Ulcerative Colitis

Cases among White Males (per 100,000 People)

Age

When ulcerative colitis is at its very worst, medication seems to be the answer. If you need medication, ask your doctor to prescribe the smallest possible amount. Also investigate possible side effects and interactions, and ask how they can be minimized.

If you have ulcerative colitis (not mucous colitis) you may have a slightly higher risk of cancer. Go for regular checkups. Should you show signs of cancer, early detection is the key to successful treatment.

A FULL LIFE DESPITE CROHN'S DISEASE

Like ulcerative colitis, Crohn's disease is an inflammatory bowel disease. But with this disease, flareups are more frequent—and totally draining, physically and mentally. Symptoms are more varied and numerous, ranging from fever and poor appetite to skin outbreaks, poor growth, delayed sexual maturity in adolescents and joint soreness. The nutritional deficiencies resulting from Crohn's disease are more severe than those caused by colitis. And because Crohn's disease burrows more deeply into the bowel wall and is more chronic, overall healing is slow.

But the severity of the disease doesn't mean it can't be tamed. To keep one step ahead of nutritional losses, you need extra vitamins and minerals. Of the various nutrients lacking in people with Crohn's disease, zinc is probably the most critical: It promotes healing, clears skin problems, sharpens sense of taste and appetite, and spurs growth and sexual maturation—all serious problems related to this disorder. When researchers at the University of Chicago measured zinc levels in 30 people with Crohn's disease, they found that zinc lagged by 39 percent in children and by 16 percent in adults, when compared with healthy people.

In another study, doctors found that seven out of ten people with Crohn's disease had a third less vitamin C in their blood than healthy people. They recommend vitamin C supplements for everyone with Crohn's disease.

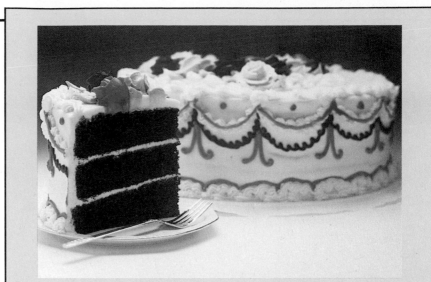

Is It an Allergy?

A number of doctors feel that many cases of ulcerative colitis may be caused by food allergy, and treating that allergy should be considered before drugs or surgery is used.

"I've found that in susceptible people, allergic reaction to commonly eaten foods is the direct cause of ulcerative colitis," says Barbara Solomon, M.D., of Baltimore, Maryland. Dr. Solomon has found that people with ulcerative colitis are always allergic to milk products and to wheat, oats, barley, rye and corn. When her patients avoid those foods (and sometimes other foods as well), the disease often improves greatly.

"Food allergy isn't the only cause of ulcerative colitis," Dr. Solomon says. "Sometimes a patient doesn't get well until I take him off tap water and have him drink only distilled water. Tap water is full of chemicals, and any one of them could be causing the problem," she adds.

Various other studies have uncovered deficiencies of vitamins B$_{12}$, A, D and K, folate, calcium, magnesium or iron in people with Crohn's disease. Consider supplements the cornerstone of your diet.

Resisting sweets also helps. Eating too much sugar may contribute to Crohn's disease, according to reports published in the *British Medical Journal*. In one survey, researchers discovered that people with Crohn's disease ate the equivalent of 10 teaspoons of sugar a day, while healthy people ate only 7. Other researchers have observed that people with Crohn's disease tend to add more sugar to their coffee, tea and breakfast cereals than others.

As with colitis, the need for dietary fiber varies in Crohn's disease, depending on the state of the intestine. If the lumen (the space inside the intestine) is very swollen, too much fiber can be harmful—stools made bulky with fiber won't be able to squeeze through. But if your lower bowel is fairly wide open, fibrous foods can help. British doctors treated 32 people with Crohn's disease with a diet rich in fiber and unrefined carbohydrates. After four years, they spent a total of only 111 days hospitalized for their disease—compared with 533 days shared by 32 Crohn's disease sufferers who did not eat a high-fiber diet.

Dietary changes offer the only real hope for relief of Crohn's disease, because medicine has very little to offer. The National Cooperative Crohn's Disease Study showed that three drugs commonly prescribed for Crohn's disease—prednisone, sulfasaluzine and azathioprine—do a poor job of relieving symptoms and preventing flareups. On the other hand, the better nourished you are, the better you can withstand flareups.

If your symptoms are life-threatening, your doctor may recommend surgery. While this step may save your life, it isn't a cure. One study revealed that, despite surgery, the disease recurred in nine out of ten people. So whatever dietary measures you take to keep the disease in check are to your advantage.

DIVERTICULITIS: THE DISEASE DIET CAN CURE

With diverticular disease, you're so constipated that your insides feel as though they've turned to stone. Yet, you're frequently surprised by bouts of diarrhea. Pain and tenderness plague the lower left side of your body, and you feel ill and feverish.

What causes all that agony?

Fruitless efforts to pass small, marblelike stools.

But let's back up a bit. Normally, large, soft stools move along the 5-foot length of your small intestine like toothpaste through a tube. Feces are nudged along gently by the circular muscles hugging the intestinal wall. However, if the feces are small and hard instead of large and soft, those muscles must push hard and long to produce any movement. Pressure builds within the intestine. Repeated episodes of strain force the intestine to balloon out at its weakest points. Those outpouchings are the cause of diverticulosis. Should the outpouchings become inflamed—as they do easily—you have diverticulitis. Feces can leak though perforations into the abdomen, poisoning your system (peritonitis). Blood vessels can burst and bleed. And after years of strain, the intestinal muscles can stiffen, trapping all stools, hard or soft. At that point, you need to be hospitalized to have your "septic system" cleaned out.

Clearly, diverticular disease is more than a simple matter of chronic constipation. Yet the solution is simple, inexpensive and as near as your pantry shelf. It's fiber. When you eat fiber, you are eating the gridwork that gives plant foods—fruits, vegetables, grain, beans, nuts—their shape. The fiber-rich coating of grains (including wheat, oats, barley, corn and rice) is called bran.

It's hard to believe that for years, doctors told people with diverticular disease to ease up on "roughage"—whole grain foods, vegetables, fruit and other high-fiber foods. Because we now know that too little fiber is what *causes* the disease. Dietary fiber absorbs water like a sponge and molds waste products into soft stools that can be passed along quickly and effortlessly. Without fiber, stools petrify and become stranded in the bowel.

Despite the simplicity of the solution, diverticulosis and diverticulitis constitute our most common intestinal disorders—especially among older people. One-third of all people over 60—and almost half of all people over age 70—have one or both forms of diverticular disease.

It's easy to see how so many people got into that fix. Since 1900, methods of processing flour and other high-fiber foods have drastically cut the average amount of dietary fiber eaten by Americans. We eat about 4 grams of fiber a day. In countries such as India, China and many parts of Africa, where food is not overly processed, people eat about 30 grams of fiber a day—and diverticular disease is practically unknown. The reason the problem doesn't show up until later years in Americans and other Westerners is that it takes 30 or 40 years of frequent bouts with constipation for the condition to develop into full-blown diverticular disease.

But it doesn't have to be that way. "Happily, we know that with diet—high-fiber diet—we can relieve, quite dramatically, over 90 percent of the symptoms of diverticular disease," says Dr. Neil S. Painter, a British physician who helped to revolutionize treatment for diverticular disease. "Already, the widespread adoption of this diet in England, for example, has reduced, quite remarkably, the need for surgery," he says.

In a British study, 75 people with diverticular disease were treated with a high-fiber diet. Over 90 percent remained symptom free for five to seven years. In another study by British doctors at the University of Oxford, 20 people who ate a high-fiber diet passed stools more quickly than 27 others who ate a low-fiber diet—and they had fewer diverticular problems. Vegetarians, who tend to eat more fruit, vegetables, seeds and whole grains than do meat eaters, average 64 percent less diverticular disease than nonvegetarians, according to a study published in the medical journal *Lancet*.

If fiber is good enough for the British, it's good enough for us. How do we put fiber back on the table?

Start by adding up to 2 table-spoons of bran a day to your cereal, fruit juice, hamburger patties, meat loaf, muffins or casseroles. The exact amount of bran you need will depend on how many other high-fiber foods you eat. But the coarser the bran, the better. A laboratory experiment by nutritionists at Cornell University showed that coarsely ground wheat bran holds more water in the feces and speeds stools along more rapidly than fine bran.

"These findings suggest that coarse bran and food products forti-fied with coarsely ground bran should be the choice of [people] with diverticular disease," stated the researchers.

The second easiest way to eat more fiber is to switch from overly refined cereals, white breads and noodles to whole grain products. Be sure to buy 100 percent whole grain bread, not so-called rye or wheat breads that contain only a small percentage of whole grain flour.

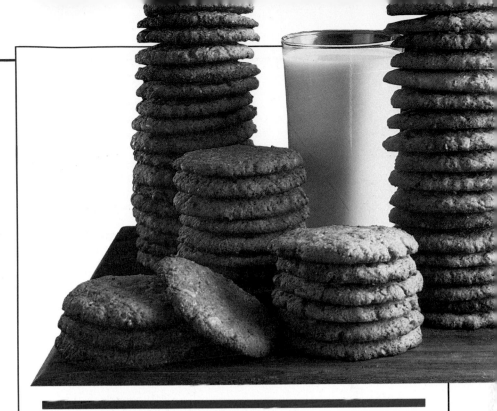

Honey Bran Cookies

Makes 2½ dozen

1 cup whole wheat pastry flour	½ cup sunflower seeds
2 teaspoons baking powder	½ cup butter
1 teaspoon cinnamon	⅓ cup honey
¾ cup bran	1 egg
	1 teaspoon vanilla

In a small bowl, sift together flour, baking powder and cinnamon. Stir in bran and sunflower seeds. In a medium mixing bowl, cream the butter and honey together until light and fluffy. Add egg and vanilla and beat well. Gradually add dry ingredients to butter mixture. From a teaspoon, drop batter onto ungreased cookie sheet. Bake in preheated 350°F oven for 10 to 12 minutes.

Fruits with edible skins, such as peaches, pears, apples, seedless grapes and berries, are fiber gold mines and make great snacks eaten out-of-hand. Or you can dice them and mix them with raisins and carrots for a waldorf-type salad. Or blend oranges, bananas and other fruit for a smooth, refreshing beverage.

For best results, you should drink plenty of water—six to eight glasses a day—on a high-fiber diet, because fiber needs water to do its job. And it's best to divide the fiber you eat among all your meals, as nature intended, rather than plunk it in all at once.

Bulk laxatives, made from seeds or seed coatings, certain vegetable gums or fibers, act like fiber in that they, too, increase the water content of stools and relieve constipation. Those products are convenient to use when you're traveling or under circumstances where you have less control than usual over what you eat. But otherwise, it's better to upgrade your entire diet with high-fiber foods than to add an expensive, fiberlike product from the drugstore.

Before you begin your new dietary regime, note this precaution. Some people with diverticulitis may not be able to eat seeds; they are not digested well and may even block the intestine. These folks should be especially wary of nuts, corn, popcorn, strawberries, raspberries, figs, grapes with seeds, poppy seeds and caraway seeds.

During a very severe attack of diverticulitis, you may be hospitalized so that you can fast safely for six or seven days to give the bowel a complete rest. Your doctor may prescribe antibiotics, if bacteria have colonized the area.

Anticholinergic drugs can reduce painful spasms during acute flareups, but used in excess they can paralyze the intestine and lead to permanent constipation. So there is some controversy as to whether those drugs should be used at all. Clearly, it's worth your while to steer clear of trouble in the first place by getting on the bran wagon for life.

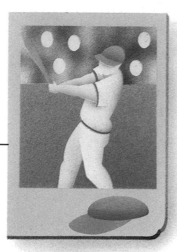

Take Me Out of the Ball Game

Hemorrhoids may have cost the Kansas City Royals the 1980 World Series—or at the very least, Game 2. George Brett, the team's star player, had developed hemorrhoids early in the season. By the end of the opening game of the Series, Brett was in excruciating pain. The Philadelphia Phillies won that game, 7-6. Brett toughed it out and tried to play Game 2, banging out 2 hits and drawing a walk before limping off the field during the 6th inning. The final score: Phillies 6, Royals 4.

Surgery saved the day, allowing Brett to help the Royals win Game 3, 4-3 and Game 4, 5-3, thus tying the Series. But in Game 5, Brett struck out in the 9th, and the Phillies won 4-3; the Philadelphia team then won the 6th game, 4-1, to take the Series championship.

NO HEMORRHOIDS, NO SURGERY

Historians say that a severe case of hemorrhoids kept Napoleon off his horse at Waterloo, delaying the battle and losing him the war.

Are you, too, losing the fight against hemorrhoids?

The pain, itching and bleeding caused by these grape-size swellings in the rectum make hemorrhoids both troublesome and embarrassing. Yet if the truth be known, many people around you share this misery.

What's at the bottom of all this? Veins in the rectum—the "holding tank" for waste—swell under pressure exerted either by straining at stool or pregnancy or both. One doctor told us that there's probably not a woman alive who, if she's had a baby, doesn't have hemorrhoids.

If you're ever to be free of the maddening itch and pain of hemorrhoids, the first thing you need is tender loving care for tender enlarged veins. A number of simple remedies can get you back in the saddle.

To avoid irritating tender anal tissues, wipe with a wet cloth instead of dry, scratchy toilet paper after a bowel movement. Avoid scented or colored paper—the fragrances and dyes can cause allergic reactions, adding fuel to the fire.

To cool and anesthetize the hot, searing pain, dab the anal area with witch hazel. Or alternate sitting on an ice pack and then in a tub of warm water.

To heal inflamed tissues, dab on wheat germ oil. It contains vitamin E, a well-known healing substance.

To relieve pain, itching and swelling even further, some people have taken bioflavonoids. They're substances found most abundantly in the white rind of citrus fruits. A doctor in Switzerland treated over 200 hemorrhoid patients with a bioflavonoid. The results, he says, were "extremely encouraging, especially where early stages of the disease are concerned. Pain and [itching] . . . often . . . disappeared entirely." Other people have found that 500 milligrams of rutin, a member of the bioflavonoid family, reduces hemorrhoidal swelling.

If your hemorrhoids itch, cut down on your intake of coffee, tea, cola, beer and chocolate. Stimulants in those foods seem to irritate the bowel.

By far, the most important strategy against hemorrhoids is to eat bran and other high-fiber foods that help to form soft stools that can be passed regularly, without strain and pain. Regular, easy bowel movements save wear and tear on existing hemorrhoids *and* prevent hemorrhoids from forming in the first place. People in rural Africa, for

example, eat plenty of vegetables, fruit, whole grains, seeds and nuts—all high in fiber. As a result, those people pass large, soft stools, and almost never have hemorrhoids.

It's never too late to benefit from fiber. First of all, fiber pushes waste out of the bowel before it forms hard, unmanageable stools that cause or inflame hemorrhoids. When nutritionists in Britain supplemented the diet of six men with 18 grams of fiber a day, the time needed to digest food in the intestine dropped from an average 67 hours—almost three days—to 42 hours—under two days.

And when people with hemorrhoids bulk up on bran, they experience less pain and bleeding with bowel movements. Danish doctors treated 51 hemorrhoid sufferers with either a fiber supplement or a look-alike placebo. After six weeks, the people who took the fiber supplement had better bowel movements and suffered far less pain and bleeding than those who did not increase their fiber intake.

Along with bran and other high-fiber foods, drink plenty of water to keep stools soft.

To reduce pressure on rectal veins during defecation, rest your heels on a small bench placed in front of the toilet. That position approximates the natural squatting position people used before the relatively

Shrink Polyps Safely

A rectal polyp is a growth that many doctors believe may signal future cancer. So it was good news when a team of doctors at West Virginia University suggested that large doses of vitamin C can obliterate polyps. They gave 9 people with rectal polyps 3,000 milligrams of vitamin C for 3 to 7 months. Polyps disappeared completely in 2 lucky people and shrank in another 3. Of the remainder, 1 was un-affected by the vitamin C and 3 dropped out of the study.

The doctors say that vitamin C apparently increases the breakdown of bile acids, which are thought to cause rectal polyps.

In a previous study, doctors gave 3,000 milligrams of vitamin C to 8 people with rectal polyps. Three had fewer polyps, and in 2 others polyps disappeared.

recent invention of the toilet.

If your hemorrhoids are beyond the help of changes in your diet or bowel habits, your doctor can remove them simply and painlessly without surgery. In a procedure called rubber band ligation, the doctor ties off the swollen veins with a rubber band. In a couple of weeks, the strangled veins

die and fall off. Because no cutting is done, you don't need general anesthesia or hospitalization, and recovery is less painful and prolonged than with hemorrhoidectomy (surgical treatment). In one study, doctors used the rubber band technique on 90 hemorrhoid sufferers with great success — most people required three or four tie-offs done at two- to four-week intervals. Few experienced pain of any kind, and no one lost time from work.

With all those possible remedies, no one should have to suffer from hemorrhoids. You may even look forward to sitting down again.

LACTOSE INTOLERANCE: MAKING FRIENDS WITH MILK

If your abdomen rumbles or feels crampy and bloated 15 to 30 minutes after you drink a glass of milk, you probably have lactose intolerance. If you experience gas or diarrhea an hour or two later, you almost certainly have the problem.

Lactose intolerance is normal and more of an inconvenience than a disease. Seventy percent of the people in the world cannot digest milk. Still, because lactose intolerance can have nutritional repercussions, there are a few things you should know about it.

Lactose is a carbohydrate compound found only in milk and milk products. In the intestines, lactose is broken down into smaller, more useful carbohydrates by lactase, an enzyme.

People are usually born with plenty of lactase. In newborns, the intestines are bustling with lactase activity, enabling them to digest large quantities of human milk. After all, that's all most babies live on for the first few months of life. Lactase activity isn't lost until the age of five or six.

Rarely, a child may be born with too little lactase. More often, the lactase activity simply diminishes with time. In the mature body, lactose is not absorbed very well. Undigested, it passes into the lower intestine, where it's fermented by bacteria, releasing carbon dioxide and hydrogen. Those gases produce gas, bloating, cramps and diarrhea.

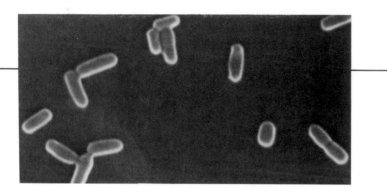

Meet the *Lactobacillus*

Many people who cannot digest milk nevertheless can enjoy certain milk products. These include yogurt and buttermilk, which can be digested with no problems. These "soured" milk products are fermented by bacteria, but not the kind of bacteria that causes colds. Instead, these products are "processed" by good bacteria, *Lactobacillus*. As the bacteria act on the milk, they digest the lactose for you. As a result, yogurt contains 40 percent less lactose than milk, while buttermilk contains about 25 percent less.

Certain cheeses, too, are ideal for people who cannot digest milk. First and foremost is cottage cheese, which contains even less lactose than fermented foods. Edam and Gouda, which are firm cheeses, contain no lactose, and hard English cheeses — cheddar and Cheshire — contain only traces.

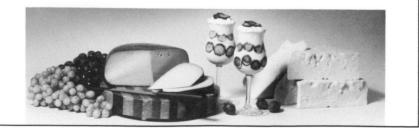

How much milk you can drink depends on how much lactase activity remains. Although some people have low lactase levels, they can still drink milk without problems (no one knows why). A person with only a slight deficiency of lactase may be able to easily digest 1 cup of milk but no more. Similarly, some people find they can tolerate small amounts of milk rationed throughout the day—but become bloated if they drink the total amount all at once.

To limit symptoms, drink milk with food, which delays the release of lactose into the intestine. If you can't tolerate any milk at all, such as the small amounts in margarine or baked goods, you may be allergic to milk rather than unable to digest it.

Because lactose intolerance occurs in varying degrees, some people may not realize they even have it until they begin to drink more milk than usual. For example, women may first notice their symptoms when they become pregnant and begin to drink milk regularly for the first time since their childhood. Others become painfully aware of the effect of milk after stomach surgery, which speeds up the emptying rate of the stomach.

If you can't drink milk, chances are your great-grandparents—and their great-grandparents—may have shared in your dilemma, depending on where in the world they originated. For example, 99 out of 100 Orientals cannot drink milk. Many blacks, American Indians, Mexicans, Jews, Italians and other ethnic groups descended from people living in Asia, Africa and southern Europe are lactose intolerant to some degree.

This inability to digest milk makes perfect sense when you consider that in practically all other land mammals, lactase activity drops off by 90 percent when breastfeeding is discontinued. In other words, lactose tolerance in adults is an aberration, and lactose intolerance is normal. Yet, some adults can digest milk. Apparently, the ability to tolerate lactose has persisted in populations that do a lot of dairy farming. Caucasians in northern and western Europe and a few pastoral tribes in Africa domesticated cows and goats between 6,000 and 10,000 years ago, and have been drinking milk ever

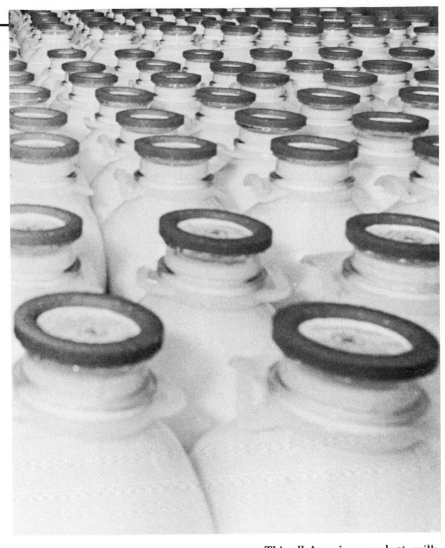

since. In most other parts of the world, milk cows were not kept and dairy foods were not dietary staples. No one knows exactly *why* people who continued to drink milk and eat dairy products could still produce lactase as adults. Nevertheless, the fact remains that those whose ancestors didn't eat a lot of dairy products usually can't tolerate lactose.

Fine, you might say. I'll just stop drinking milk. But the solution to one problem poses another. Dairy products are unmatched as concentrated sources of calcium. Growing children, adolescents, pregnant women and nursing mothers need all the calcium they can get—1,200 milligrams a day, the amount in 1 quart of milk. Women in general tend to develop the weak, brittle bones of osteoporosis after menopause if they get too little calcium. They need up to 1,600 milligrams of calcium a day. Yet many older women have too little lactase to handle more than a few

This all-American product, milk, may be just that—American. Or at least northern European. There are many places in the world where people are lactose intolerant and can't drink milk. In those areas, dairy farming was unknown until recently or milk and milk products make up only a small part of the total diet. In the U.S., many people whose ancestors originated in those areas, and native Indians, cannot drink fresh milk, either. Some estimates say that only 30 percent of the world's population can drink milk without difficulty. Most of them are northern Europeans or their descendants.

ounces of milk a day—hardly enough to protect their bones.

You can get around lactose intolerance without shortchanging yourself on calcium. Most lactose intolerant people can produce some lactase, even if it's only a trickle. Therefore, it's possible to drink modest amounts of low-fat milk without provoking symptoms.

If you can drink any milk at all, be sure it's fortified with vitamin D, which stimulates intestinal absorption of calcium and helps to ensure that you use the calcium you get. If milk is out of the question, try to get out in the sunshine, the chief source of vitamin D. Fish and fish-liver oils also contribute this vitamin.

To help you tolerate milk, you can also buy a commercial enzyme product called Lact-Aid. One packet of the powdered lactase added to a quart of milk predigests the lactose for you. Lact-Aid is sold in pharmacies, some supermarkets and health food stores. Or you can buy milk commercially treated with the enzyme.

Beyond that, calcium supplements are the ultimate insurance against a deficiency. Your best bets are calcium gluconate and calcium carbonate. But avoid calcium lactate, which contains lactose and may provoke symptoms.

Lactose intolerance doesn't have to cramp your nutritional style. By making a few simple changes in your diet, you can easily compensate for the condition.

APPENDICITIS: DON'T BE TAKEN BY SURPRISE

If you're like most people, you probably assume that appendicitis strikes out of the blue, with no provocation. But you'd be assuming wrong.

A second belief, that a watermelon seed or other foreign body can cause an attack of appendicitis, also is highly questionable. Appendicitis primarily results from pebbles of feces that irritate and contaminate the organ—a wormlike outpouching along the first stretch of the large intestine. Because it has a small opening and no exit, it's an all-too-convenient niche for collecting feces.

Although only 3 to 6 inches long and ⅓ inch in diameter, once inflamed an appendix can swell to eight to ten times its normal size.

But a surprise attack of appendicitis is not really a surprise at all. Several years ago, Denis P. Burkitt, M.D.—a British doctor who linked hemorrhoids to a low-fiber diet—proposed that passing small, hard stools also inflames the appendix. In short, a low-fiber diet sets the stage for appendicitis. According to Dr. Burkitt, small stools increase pressure in the colon and the appendix. Straining to pass them further raises pressure throughout the abdomen. Eating whole grain foods and other sources of fiber allows formation of large, soft stools that are passed easily and do not stress the colon.

A scientist in Sweden, Einar Arnbjörnsson, of the University of Lund, decided to test Dr. Burkitt's hypothesis by comparing the food intake of 31 patients with acute appendicitis with that of 30 healthy people who served as controls.

After evaluating the seven-day food diaries of all 61 people in the experiment, Dr. Arnbjörnsson found that the problem-free folks ate an average of 21 grams of fiber, while those with appendicitis ate an average of 17.4 grams—a small but significant difference. Even more impressive was the fact that only 16 percent of the persons in the group with appendicitis consumed more than 25 grams of fiber per day, reported the doctor, while 43 percent of the control group had eaten that amount.

RECOVERING FROM AN APPENDECTOMY

If you suspect that you or your child is having an attack of appendicitis, call a doctor. Appendicitis rarely, if ever, subsides by itself. Left alone, the appendix will burst, spreading the infection into the abdomen, causing a potentially fatal condition. An inflamed appendix must be drained and removed—and the sooner, the better.

Because the appendix serves no purpose, you won't miss it when it's gone. How quickly you recover depends on whether or not your

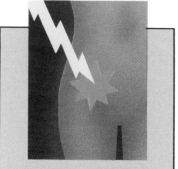

Appendicitis Alert

Appendicitis pain usually strikes abruptly, with cramps throughout the abdomen, nausea, vomiting and a slight fever.

Within 6 to 18 hours, the pain zeros in on the lower right abdomen. The victim is usually constipated and has little or no appetite.

Call a doctor if any pain in the abdomen persists for more than a few hours, especially if the pain is accompanied by any of the symptoms described above.

appendix has ruptured. The average hospital stay is one week, but after a rupture, expect a stay of two weeks or longer. If your appendix hasn't burst, you'll be able to get out of bed the day after surgery. Otherwise, you'll be bedridden for a few days.

To rest the intestinal tract, you won't be able to eat or drink for a day or two. When you do resume a regular diet, though, add a tablespoon or two of bran to your cereal or other food. This fiber not only prevents constipation, but also helps to prevent blood clots in the veins of the legs, a common and potentially serious problem in people who are confined to bed.

It takes a week or more for the incision to heal, but you can speed healing by taking the nutrients crucial to successful healing, vitamins A and C and zinc. Vitamin C is essential for the manufacture of collagen, a tough, fibrous substance that gives strength to new tissue by cementing cells together. Vitamin C also heals wounds indirectly by encouraging tiny blood vessels called capillaries to renew themselves in the wound area, bringing with them red blood cells, nutrients and antibodies that fight infectious bacteria. This renewal is especially critical after an appendectomy, because the infected organ is removed through the incision, making the surgical wound particularly susceptible to infection. The minimum dose of vitamin C required for wound healing is 500 milligrams a day.

Just as vitamin C sparks collagen formation, vitamin A influences the rate at which the collagen is laid down between cells, and so it, too, encourages the growth and repair of tissues. The addition of supplemental amounts of vitamin A to the diet has been shown to enhance the process of wound healing. Doses of 10,000 I.U. a day meet the approximate needs of surgical patients.

Zinc plays a pivotal role in wound healing because it sparks the release of vitamin A from the liver and enhances that vitamin's role in healing. Zinc also is fundamental to production of new cells, metabolism of protein for tissue repair and infection control. One study found that surgical patients given a zinc-

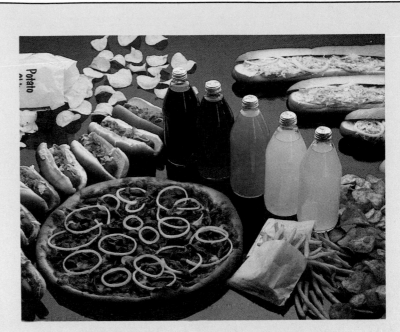

Saturday Night Feeder

Weekend gorging may cause more than just a case of Monday morning indigestion—it also may contribute to attacks of appendicitis early in the week.

That's the theory of Lloyd Roberts, M.D. This Maine pathologist discovered that hospital admissions for acute appendicitis peaked on Sunday, Monday and Tuesday, then fell off during the rest of the week.

He reviewed the cases of 137 people treated for appendicitis at the Penobscot Bay Medical Center in Rockland, Maine, for almost 2 years. The first 3 days of the week averaged 23.3 admissions, compared with 16.5 for the rest of the week.

Appendicitis has an incubation period of a few hours to several days. That leads Dr. Roberts to suspect that there's "clearly something about the weekend" that increases susceptibility to or causes the condition. He cites eating, drinking, exercising, outdoor exposure, television watching, sex and sleeping as the chief weekend overindulgences. However, he singles out "dietary excess" as the most likely culprit in appendicitis.

supplemented diet had pinker, cleaner, healthier-looking new tissues and more rapidly healing wounds than those who did not. Thirty milligrams of zinc a day is necessary to ensure optimum wound healing.

Vitamin E oil, applied to the incision, can reduce the pain, redness and itch of the appendectomy scar.

By taking the recommended steps to speed your recovery, you can help make this crisis as uneventful as possible.

CYSTITIS: SIMPLE WAYS TO PURGE THE GERMS

Urination is something you take for granted—until the urine burns like iodine on a raw wound. Or until you feel like you have to "go" right after you've just "gone." Your abdomen and back ache. You may even pass a drop or two of blood.

Cystitis, a urinary tract infection, affects millions of people—mostly women. And it's generally not a once-in-a-lifetime experience. In 80 percent of those who get cystitis, the infection returns again and again. Each time, they're awakened several times a night by the urge to urinate. They run to the bathroom every 20 minutes at work, and often are in too much pain to concentrate on their jobs. On a personal level, they no longer enjoy sexual relations.

Cystitis may be caused by any of various organisms, including *Trichomonas* and *Chlamydia*. The most common cause, though, is *Escherichia coli* bacteria, which normally live in the large intestine and the rectum without causing any trouble. If those bacteria find their way into the urethra—the 1½-inch-long tube leading to the bladder and kidneys—the resulting infection makes urination urgent, frequent and painful. Should the infection spread to the kidney—a rare occurrence—it can do serious damage.

Certainly it's only a tiny trip from the rectum to the urethra, but certain habits make that trip even easier for bacteria to take. Sexual activity seems to trigger recurrent cystitis in most women. The theory is that intercourse pushes bacteria from the area of the urethra into the bladder. Simply washing before and after sex helps to sanitize the area and prevent infection. Another preventive measure is to urinate within 10 minutes after sex, thus flushing bacteria and other organisms out of the urethra before they have a chance to do their dirty work.

PREVENTIVE HYGIENE

Still, women of all ages, from little girls to elderly widows, get cystitis, so there's clearly more to recurrent cystitis than sex. Wiping from back to front after you use the toilet drags rectal bacteria into the urethral opening. The reverse—wiping from front to back—prevents that. ("Wipe down, not up" is the way one three-year-old was taught—proving that little girls can learn preventive hygiene early in life.)

No matter how busy you are, don't hold your urine indefinitely after feeling the urge. Ignoring nature's call distends the bladder wall, making it more susceptible to infection. And when urine accumulates in the bladder, so does bacteria. An empty bladder is less readily infected.

Wearing loose clothing and cotton underwear also helps to prevent cystitis. Tight jeans, girdles, pantyhose and nylon briefs "hermetically seal" and irritate the urethral area, contributing to the growth of bacteria.

Women are especially prone to cystitis during pregnancy, particularly during the last three months. At that time, organs are crowded together. Scrunched between the womb and the pubic bone, the bladder may not be able to empty completely. Bacteria lingering in leftover urine become fruitful and multiply. During pregnancy, it's especially important to take precautions against cystitis, because hormonal changes at that time seem to encourage susceptibility. Women using a diaphragm for birth control may find it increases susceptibility to infection. The device's rim can push against the neck of the bladder, preventing complete urination. Changing to either a slightly smaller diaphragm or another method of birth control prevented further bouts of cystitis in 98.4 percent of women studied by Larrian Gillespie, M.D., a urologist and clinical instructor at the University of California at Irvine.

HOME DETECTION

You don't necessarily need an elaborate urologic workup of lab tests and

Symptoms of Cystitis

According to Larrian Gillespie, M.D., the signs of cystitis are easy to recognize:
• The urgent need to urinate often;
• Sharp stinging during urination, often accompanied by a gnawing pain in the lower abdomen;
• Occasionally, blood in the urine;
• Feeling that the bladder is full after urination.

Recognizing the illness can hasten relief of cystitis.

X rays to tell if you have a simple urinary infection. Calvin M. Kunin, M.D., of the Ohio State University Medical School, has developed a home test kit that women can use regularly to detect infections before they become painful. The kit (MICROSTIX-Nitrite, by Ames) is especially useful to people who are prone to repeated infections despite their best efforts at prevention.

To test for the presence of bacteria, dip a test stick into freshly voided morning urine and compare it to a color chart printed on the packet. If the test stick turns pink, indicating an infection is present, you should take steps to purge the germs from your urinary tract.

At the first sign of cystitis, drink lots of water—eight glasses a day. It flushes bacteria out of the urinary tract and dilutes the urine, thus relieving the burning of urination.

You can substitute cranberry juice for some of that water. No other juice contains hippuric acid, unique in that it inhibits bacterial growth. In fact, some folks find that fresh cranberries ground up and mixed with plain yogurt work better than the juice. One woman who had suffered with cystitis for most of her life said, "It is just a year since I last took any medication for bladder infection and a year since I've been free from it. This after 40 years of this scourge!

"Nothing ever really helped for long. Canned cranberry juice did nothing. But this is what helped: I ground up fresh cranberries in the food chopper and mixed this with enough honey to make it palatable. At the first indication of trouble, I started eating it with plain yogurt. The last full siege I had, the kind that hits within an hour, symptoms were greatly relieved in 6 hours and completely gone in 12. No medications," she said.

Extra vitamin C also helps to battle cystitis, by killing bacteria.

Avoiding Those Cystitis Traps

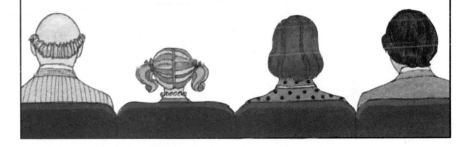

Ignoring the urge to urinate is a major cause of cystitis. Watching long movies, videotaped programs and pay movie stations on television—those with no commercial breaks—contributes to cystitis by not providing opportunities to go to the bathroom. So do long auto trips. People often delay urination because restrooms are hard to find in today's huge shopping malls; because they fear contracting venereal disease in public toilets; because of the bother of removing neck-to-thigh foundation garments; because of embarrassment at leaving the room at social events; and because of being too busy with their housework or job.

While the body naturally concentrates vitamin C in the urine, large doses—500 to 1,000 milligrams over the course of a day—help to saturate the urinary tract with the vitamin, helping to wipe out *E. coli* bacteria.

Avoid coffee, tea, alcohol and spicy foods during a cystitis attack. They may irritate an already-sensitive urinary tract.

If your symptoms don't subside within 24 hours, call your doctor. Stubborn cases may not respond without antibiotics or other medication.

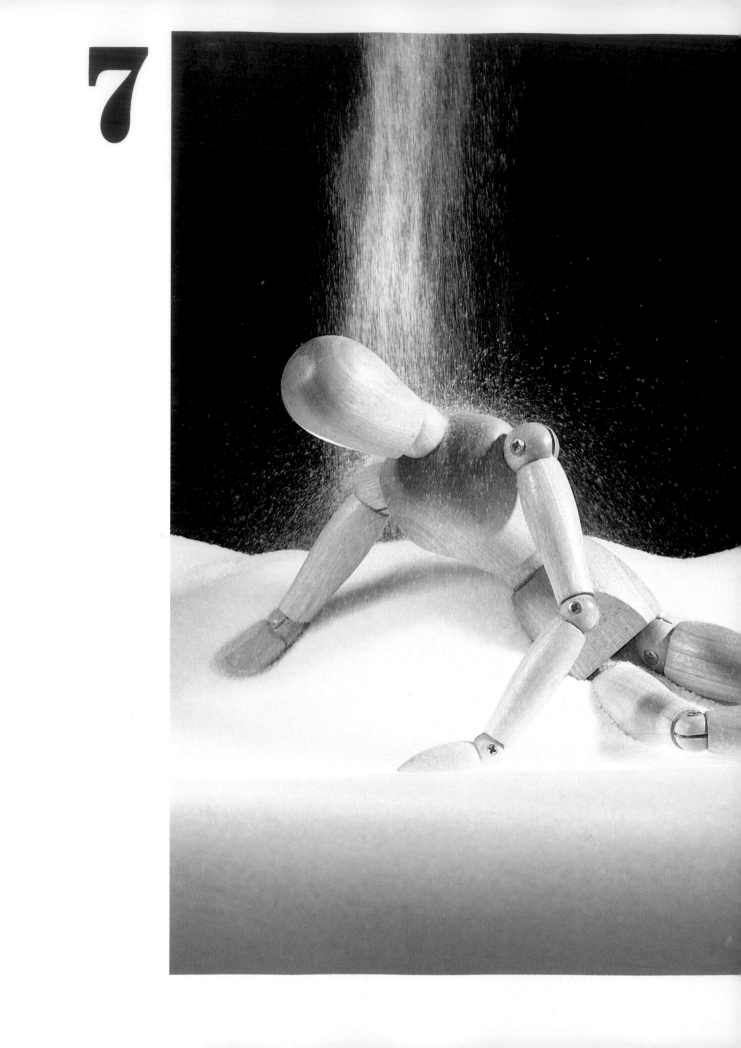

7

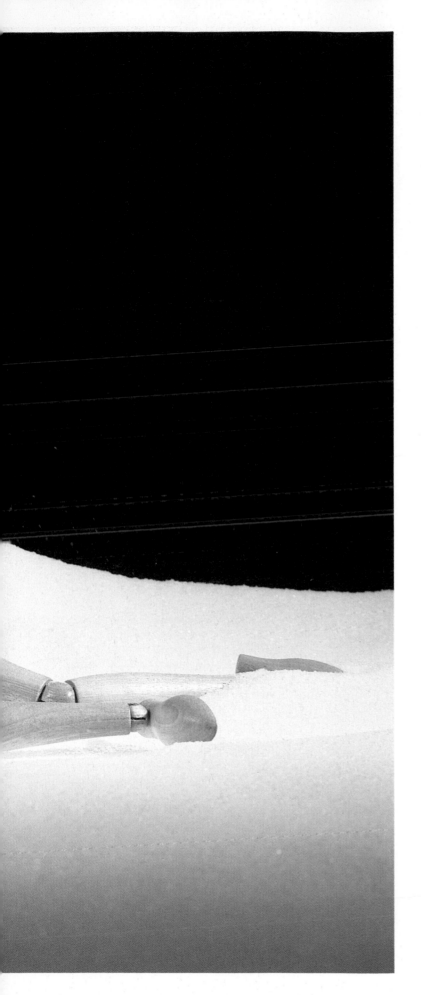

Diabetes: The Sugar Disease

Insulin isn't the *whole* answer. Along with medication, don't overlook the benefits of fiber-rich foods and exercise.

Diabetes has confounded the modern medical establishment. They thought they had it licked back in the 1920s when insulin was first used as a treatment. No such luck. Diabetes is still with us, and stronger than ever.

There are many reasons, but perhaps the least obvious is that we have been so busy developing complicated medical treatments that we may have missed some approaches that are less high-tech and a bit more natural. In the medical journals, you can read about the subcutaneous insulin infusion pump, or the siliconized needle, or maybe monocomponent insulins or multiple injection therapy. Pretty heady stuff. Only a highly advanced technology could come up with all that gear. You'd expect a big payoff. You'd be disappointed.

Lawrence Power, M.D., professor of medicine at Wayne State University and director of the Metabolic Center in Southfield, Michigan, measured the effects of these high-tech advances in diabetic care. The improvement in blood sugar concentrations in a group of diabetic patients over the period 1969-1979 was 1 percent. Dr. Power's feelings? "Chagrin."

Indeed, the recent history of diabetes is nothing to smile about. The incidence of diabetes—to say nothing of the attendant complications of blindness, gum disease and gangrene—has increased tenfold since the 1930s. With the disease claiming 6 percent more people each year than the year before, things are getting worse.

Worse in the United States, that is. But not in Africa or Japan or anywhere where people are still eating simpler diets rich in complex carbohydrates and high-fiber foods. At one point, scientists thought that the low incidence of diabetes in those groups might be genetic. Yet when Africans and Japanese move to the United States and acquire Western eating habits, they promptly acquire the American incidence of diabetes.

Other evidence has been piling up for years. And it's hard to ignore. Take wartime Britain. The number of deaths from diabetes dropped 55 percent for men and 54 percent for women. The reason? Some medical experts say it was the coarse "poor man's" black bread that replaced highly refined, processed white bread.

Medical researchers are finding that what's true of high-fiber foods may be equally true of other natural treatments like regular exercise and food supplements. Even such staid medical societies as the British and American diabetes associations have changed their tune about methods of treatment.

The consensus, slowly emerging from doctors and researchers, is that *you* can manage or prevent diabetes.

"In affluent societies...most diabetes is preventable," says Kelly West, M.D., who was involved with a massive worldwide study of diabetes coordinated by the World Health Organization. But before we find out how to prevent or treat this disease, let's find out exactly what it is. And to know that, we have to look at how your body regulates blood sugar.

THE BLOOD SUGAR STORY

When you digest a meal, the carbohydrates in the food you just ate are turned into glucose. This simple sugar, your body's prime source of energy, pours into the bloodstream to be carried throughout your body. Some of this blood sugar is taken up immediately—by your brain, which requires a constant supply, and by other cells that need energy right away. But much is packed away for future use, stored in the liver and muscles as a starch called glycogen, or in adipose tissue as fat. If, for example, you go for a long walk two hours after lunch, some of the glycogen will be turned back into glucose to supply energy.

It is vital that the level of sugar in your blood stays relatively even: too little would starve the cells of energy, and too much would disrupt the body's chemical balance. The key to this regulation is insulin, a hormone secreted by the pancreas. Insulin makes it easier for glucose to enter the cells for energy, and to be stored in liver, muscle and fat cells for later use. Insulin also controls the rate at which the liver produces and releases glucose. A major problem in diabetes is an excessive release of glucose from the liver. Normally, insulin would control this. But if there is not enough insulin, glucose builds up in the bloodstream and the result is diabetes.

Actually, there are two types of diabetes. If your pancreas can manufacture virtually no insulin, you will suffer from the more severe type, often called insulin-dependent diabetes. Children frequently have this type, so it's also called juvenile diabetes. If you have adult-onset diabetes—by far the most common

Since 1935, the incidence of diabetes has increased more than sixfold. Obesity and the standard diet play a key role in the development of this disease. We know that in this century, our consumption of refined foods has increased, while our fiber intake has declined—both factors that disturb blood sugar control.

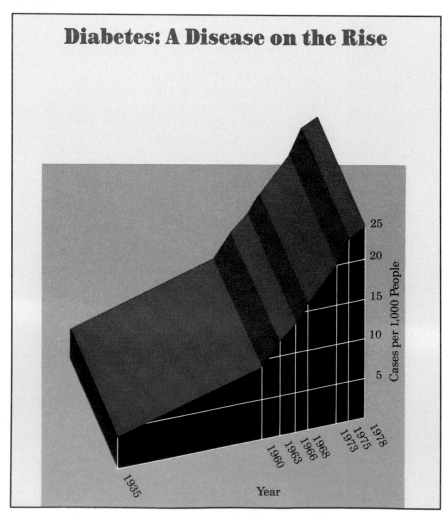

Diabetes: A Disease on the Rise

Cases per 1,000 People

25
20
15
10
5

1935 1960 1963 1966 1968 1973 1975 1978

Year

variety—even though your supply of insulin is about right, it is not put to proper use and therefore does not meet the body's needs.

A DIET FOR DIABETES

In the past, diabetics had to watch their diet with a mental microscope—too many carbohydrates, they were told, would push their blood sugar into the danger zone. Today, it's a lot easier. As easy as eating an apple or a baked potato, and not making a habit of roast beef and cheesecake. But aren't apples and potatoes carbohydrates? Isn't that the type of food diabetics are supposed to *avoid*? Not any more.

It's true that until recently the medical establishment thought the best way to fight diabetes was to cut out all carbohydrates—the sugars and starches. The body breaks them down into glucose. If the body has trouble handling glucose, the thinking went, then don't give it any kind of sugar, simple or complex. So out went the refined sugars and starches like jelly and maple syrup and white bread, and right along with them went complex carbohydrates like noodles, potatoes and brown rice. But in 1979 the American Diabetes Association (ADA), which had recommended the low-carbohydrate diet for decades, finally saw the error of its ways. In a special report—"Principals of Nutrition and Dietary Recommendations for Individuals with Diabetes Mellitus"—the ADA stated that foods high in dietary fiber are desirable in diabetic meal plans. And in England, the British Diabetic Association issued a statement saying that "a lowered fat, increased carbohydrate, high-fiber diet is recommended for all diabetics."

Why the switch?

It was caused by studies like those conducted by James Anderson, M.D., and his associates at the University of Kentucky College of Medicine in Lexington.

THE FIBER FACTOR

In one experiment conducted by Dr. Anderson, 20 adult-onset diabetics were fed the standard low-carbohydrate diet for about a week, during which

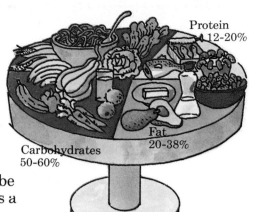

Pregnancy: A Safe and Healthy Diet

A diabetic pregnancy is cause for real concern. However, with proper care, it can be about as healthy as a normal pregnancy. According to Richard L. Byyny, M.D., a professor of medicine at the University of Colorado, the diabetic mother who maintains strict blood glucose control at low levels is at just slightly greater risk of stillborn birth than a healthy pregnant woman. To keep these levels low, Barbara Jacobs, a nutritionist at the Hospital of the University of Pennsylvania, believes a diet higher in fiber may be a key factor. The rule of thumb, according to Ms. Jacobs, is sticking to a diet high in fiber and low in fat, and gaining only about 22 to 30 pounds during the total pregnancy.

"But the first and the most important thing," says Ms. Jacobs, "is to be under proper medical supervision, counseled by a registered nutritionist and managed by a doctor, because each case can be different."

Protein 12-20%
Fat 20-38%
Carbohydrates 50-60%

time their insulin doses averaged 26 units a day. Then they switched to a diet high in carbohydrates and fiber.

"On the high-carbohydrate, high-fiber diets there was a rapid drop in insulin requirements," Dr. Anderson says. "Insulin shots could be completely discontinued in eight patients.

"At the completion of the high-carbohydrate, high-fiber diets, insulin doses, which averaged 11 units per day, were less than half of those required on the standard diabetic diets. Despite lower insulin doses, blood sugars were about 20 points lower. Thus these diets lowered insulin requirements and led to improvement in blood sugar."

When Dr. Anderson used the high-fiber diet to treat 42 adult-onset diabetics at the Veterans' Medical Center in Lexington, the results were *(continued on page 108)*

Diabetes and Dining Out

Many people with diabetes hesitate to eat in restaurants. And, indeed, it *is* easier to control what's in your diet when you prepare your food at home. However, a fairly good—and safe—meal can be had in a restaurant.

It often helps to explain to the waiter or waitress that you have special food requirements. Ask if dishes additional to those on the printed menu are available. Moreover, feel free to question cooking methods. Is the fish broiled or fried? If fried, how much oil is used and what kind? Are fresh fruits available for dessert? Can you make substitutions in side dishes?

By making polite requests, the person with diabetes often can dine both safely and in sumptuous elegance. *Bon appétit!*

The diabetic need not fear dining out. The trick is to select wisely from the menu. Here, for instance, is an elegant meal that is entirely acceptable in the diabetic diet. For an appetizer, tomato juice followed by a fresh garden salad lightly dressed with yogurt-herb dressing. The entree consists of broiled flounder accompanied by green beans, mushrooms and a whole wheat roll. For dessert, delicious poached pears, with herb tea to drink.

Exchanging Foods (Restaurant Style)

Six of one, a half dozen of another. Some foods are equal exchanges in a diabetic menu, which should be developed with your physician or dietician. Generally, foods are divided into six broad groups: milk, vegetables, fruits, bread, meat and fat. You can exchange any food in one group for any other food in that same group. Specific amounts are listed in the chart below.

Milk	Vegetables—continued	Fruits—continued	Fruits—continued	Breads—continued	Fat
Food/Portion	Food/Portion	Food/Portion	Food/Portion	Food/Portion	Food/Portion
Skim milk, 1 cup	Celery, ½ cup	Blueberries, ½ cup	Tangerine, 1 medium	Lima beans, ⅓ cup	Avocado, ⅛ large
Yogurt made from skim milk (plain), 1 cup	Eggplant, ½ cup	Figs, dried, 1	**Breads**	Peas, green, ½ cup	Olives, 5 small
1% fat, fortified milk, 1 cup	Green pepper, ½ cup	Grapefruit, ½ medium	Food/Portion	Potato, ½ cup	Peanuts, 20 whole
2% fat, fortified milk, 1 cup	Mushrooms, ½ cup	Grapes, 12	Whole wheat, 1 slice	Sweet potato, ¼ cup	Walnuts, 6 small
Yogurt made from 2% fat, fortified milk (plain), 1 cup	Onions, ½ cup	Honeydew, ⅛ medium	Pumpernickel or rye, 1 slice	**Meats**	Nuts, other, 6 small
	Rhubarb, ½ cup	Mango, ½ small	Raisin, 1 slice	Food/Portion	Margarine (regular stick), 1 tsp.
Whole milk, 1 cup	String beans, ½ cup	Nectarine, 1 small	Biscuit, 1	Lean beef, 1 oz.	Mayonnaise, 1 tsp.
Buttermilk, 1 cup	Tomatoes, ½ cup	Orange, 1 small	English muffin, ½ small	Lamb, 1 oz.	Butter, 1 tsp.
Yogurt (plain), 1 cup	Tomato juice, ½ cup	Peach, 1 medium	Pork, 1 oz.	Bacon, 1 strip
	Turnips, ½ cup	Pear, 1 small	Plain roll, 1	Veal, 1 oz.	Sour cream, 2 tbsp.
Vegetables		Pineapple, ½ cup	Tortilla, 1	Poultry, 1 oz.	Heavy cream, 1 tbsp.
Food/Portion	**Fruits**	Prunes, 2 medium	Rice (cooked), ½ cup	Fish, 1 oz.	Cream cheese, 1 tbsp.
	Food/Portion	Raisins, 2 tablespoons	Pasta (cooked), ½ cup	Cottage cheese, ¼ cup	Oil (dressing), 1 tbsp.
Asparagus, ½ cup		Strawberries, ¾ cup	Corn, ⅓ cup	Egg, 1	
Cabbage, ½ cup	Apple, 1 small			Duck, 1 oz.	
Carrots, ½ cup	Banana, ½ small				

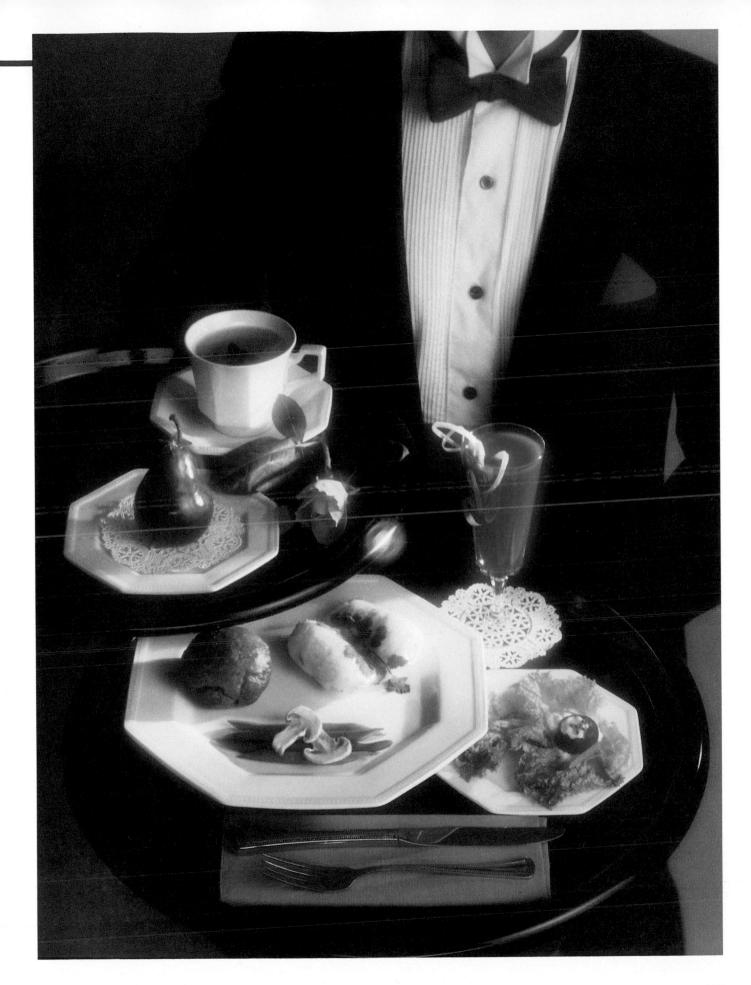

much the same. Twelve of the patients did not use insulin injections but took drugs that stimulate the pancreas to produce more insulin. While on the diet, 10 of the 12 were taken off the drugs completely, and 2 were able to substantially reduce their doses. Of the 18 patients who were using low doses of insulin (between 14 and 20 units a day), 16 were able to quit insulin completely. Of the 12 patients receiving moderate doses, 5 were also able to abandon the shots.

Dr. Anderson also treated a group of six juvenile diabetics who were receiving over 40 units of insulin a day. While none of those patients was able to discontinue their insulin shots when they switched to a high-fiber, high-carbohydrate diet, all of them required less insulin than before. In some cases, juvenile diabetics totally dependent on outside

Sugar Substitutes: The Real Scoop

Because diabetics have problems using sugar, artificial sweeteners seem to be a tempting alternative. But sugar substitutes present other problems, many of which are ill-defined.

Saccharin may cause cancer. Saccharin may not cause cancer. Fructose, the super-sweet fruit sugar, is more easily metabolized by the cells and is better for diabetics. Fructose isn't more easily metabolized by the cells and isn't better for diabetics. Sorbitol is safe. Sorbitol isn't. Cyclamates were banned in 1970. Cyclamates were no worse than saccharin, which wasn't banned. And so on.

Adding to the confusion about sugar substitutes is a new product called aspartame. Some 180 times sweeter than sugar, it is made of 2 natural proteins, which means that diabetics can metabolize it without insulin.

But aspartame is not without problems, either. John Olney, M.D., of the Washington University School of Medicine in St. Louis, did studies with laboratory rats suggesting that aspartame might cause brain damage. Richard Wurtman, Ph.D., a neuroendocrinologist at MIT, has suggested that the combination of aspartame with other foods might cause chemicals in the brain to change, which in turn could affect behavior.

Even if these researchers are wrong about aspartame, its use still raises some tough questions. Say it replaces the 8 teaspoons of sugar in each of the 419 12-ounce cans of pop that the average American drinks. Do we want to go on encouraging the consumption of 39 gallons a year of soda pop, whether sugared or sugar free, by either diabetics or nondiabetics?

insulin were able to reduce their intake by 25 percent.

Why does a diet rich in complex carbohydrates and fiber work so well? First, complex carbohydrates take longer to break down into glucose. And according to Dr. Anderson, the fiber slows that breakdown even more.

"After you eat a meal, there is a big pulse of carbohydrates entering the system," he says. "Fiber slows the absorption so there is a gradual release of it into the body."

Other scientists have added fiber supplements to otherwise normal diets, and recorded significantly lower blood sugar and reduced need for insulin. But Dr. Anderson contends that the best results are obtained when the patient's *entire* diet is altered.

TOO MUCH FAT

A doctor who has followed Dr. Anderson's lead is Julian Whitaker, M.D., of Huntington, California. But he believes that while the ADA diet is an improvement, the amount of fat it allows — a maximum of 34 percent of all calories — is still too high.

"The typical American diet derives 42 percent of its calories from fat," Dr. Whitaker says. "You could say there's obviously something wrong with that for the simple reason that natural foods, the kind we have always eaten until this present age, don't have anywhere near that much fat in them. Even more important, when we put diabetic patients on a high-carbohydrate, high-fiber, low-fat diet, nearly all of them are able to reduce their requirement for insulin, and many, particularly patients with adult-onset diabetes, are able to give up insulin altogether.

"The real enemy of the diabetic is fat. Fat actually tends to block the natural action of insulin," Dr. Whitaker claims.

It's not surprising that a low-fat, high-fiber diet cuts cholesterol, a promoter of heart disease in all people, but especially in diabetics. Dr. Anderson reports an average drop of 30 percent in cholesterol levels in his patients' blood. Taken along with reductions in insulin requirements —

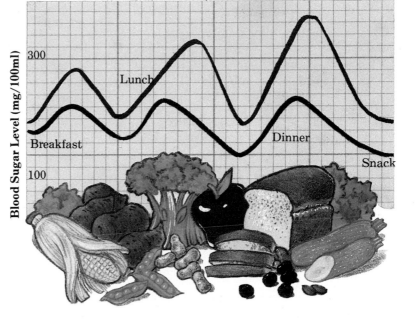

Blood Sugar of Diabetics on Low- and High-Fiber Diets

Blood Sugar Level (mg/100ml)

300

Lunch

Breakfast

100

Dinner

Snack

The red line on this graph represents fluctuations of blood sugar levels for a person eating a low-fiber diet. The blue line represents the significantly lower levels of someone on a high-fiber diet.

some reductions as high as 60 percent — you're talking strong heart, clear eyes, sound feet, you name it. Wherever blood goes, and that's everywhere, the body is healthier.

Cutting a diabetic's intake of fat has still another advantage. Weight control.

If diabetics weren't fat, they probably wouldn't be diabetics — at least not adult-onset diabetics. Over 80 percent of diabetics are overweight. Their livers, muscles and fat cells become insensitive to insulin. The pancreas, exhausted from making enough insulin to handle all the food stuffed into the digestive system, finally takes time off from the job. The result is a buildup of glucose in the blood. That means diabetes and eventually shots and pills from your doctor.

Weight loss can reverse the process.

"If early in diabetes a person loses weight and keeps it off — the disease may never come back," says Dr. Kelly West.

SUPPLEMENTS FOR DIABETICS

A diet high in fiber-rich foods and low in fat is brimming with vitamins and minerals. But doctors have found that extra doses of nutrients taken in supplement form can also help treat diabetes. Let's review those supplements one by one.

Vitamin E. Marvin L. Bierenbaum, M.D., of the Atherosclerosis Research Group in Montclair, New Jersey, found that vitamin E lowers the amount of sugar in the blood.

When Dr. Bierenbaum gave 2,000 I.U. of vitamin E per day for six weeks to a group of 25 diabetics, their blood sugar levels fell by 6 percent, a change significant enough to make him announce his findings at the American Heart Association

Convention in Washington, D.C. (The levels of vitamin E used in Dr. Bierenbaum's study should be taken only under the supervision of your doctor.)

Chromium. Another dietary factor that apparently makes a difference in the management of diabetes is called GTF, or glucose tolerance factor. Scientists discovered that nutrient when they found that rats having problems with sugar metabolism were helped when brewer's yeast was added to their diets. Researchers isolated the substance in the yeast that was causing the improvement, and determined that its main ingredient was the trace mineral chromium. Chromium is linked to a combination of niacin and amino acids in a way that makes the chromium more active in the body. Chromium appears to increase the effectiveness of the body's insulin in regulating blood sugar levels.

Chromium's benefits apply to humans as well as rats. In one demonstration of that fact, scientists at Columbia University worked with elderly people, some of them diabetic and some of them not. The volunteers were fed either chromium-rich brewer's yeast or chromium-poor torula yeast as a supplement to their diet. The brewer's yeast improved sugar metabolism, not just in the diabetic patients, but in all the people tested.

"Chromium-rich brewer's yeast improved glucose tolerance and cholesterol in elderly normal and diabetic subjects, while chromium-poor torula yeast did not," the researchers said. "An improvement in insulin sensitivity also occurred with chromium supplementation."

We know that the total amount of chromium in the body decreases as people get older, just as they become more and more susceptible to diabetes. Brewer's yeast, rich in chromium, might very well *prevent* diabetes in older people, as well as helping people who already have the disease.

Vitamin B₆. At the Thordek Medical Center in Chicago, diabetics with neuropathy (nerve degeneration) and signs of vitamin B₆ deficiency were

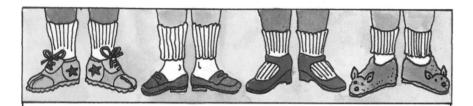

Special Care of the Feet

Diabetics are especially prone to circulatory problems, and since your feet are farthest from your heart, they're likely to suffer more than the rest of your body. Because poor circulation promotes infection, which in turn raises blood glucose levels, diabetics should consider any break in the skin serious enough to consult a doctor.

Here's how to prevent problems from developing. Keep your feet scrupulously clean and dry. Always wear clean socks. Keep toenails trimmed straight across, level with the tops of your toes, to avoid ingrown toenails. Avoid excessive heat or hot water—you could unwittingly burn your feet, since impaired circulation dulls foot sensation. Be careful not to impede circulation—don't sit cross-legged or wear tight shoes, stockings or garters. Inspect your feet daily. If you find any cracks, cuts, punctures or bruises, don't treat them yourself. If your feet become infected, your doctor should determine whether you need extra insulin.

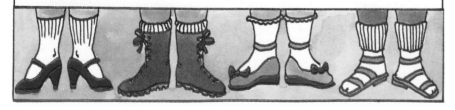

given B_6 supplements. At the conclusion of the testing, symptoms like pain, burning and numbness were either greatly reduced or completely gone.

Myoinositol. Myoinositol, a compound related to the B vitamins, also may be involved in preventing the nerve damage that often causes pain, numbness and impotence in diabetics. After clinical trials with 15 patients, Rex S. Clements, M.D., director of the clinical research center at the University of Alabama Hospitals, reported "a statistically significant improvement in nerve function on the high-myoinositol diet."

Sources of myoinositol are not hard to find—particularly among high-fiber, high-carbohydrate natural foods. They include cantaloupes, citrus fruits, peanuts and whole grains.

There may never be a last word in preventing diabetes. But the research on the disease has started to change from seeking one-word answers—like insulin—to striking the balance of natural diet, exercise and self-care. It may not be as "advanced" as high-tech medicine, but it works.

EXERCISE IS A MUST

But diet and supplements aren't the only natural treatments for diabetes. Exercise helps, too.

Vijay R. Soman, M.D., and his colleagues at Yale University, studied the effects of physical training on six healthy but sedentary men. They exercised four times a week for six weeks. After the six weeks, Dr. Soman found that the men's average "sugar uptake by insulin" was 30 percent higher—in other words, their ability to regulate blood sugar was much more effective. He also tested each person's fitness level and found that the fitter the man, the less he showed a tendency to develop diabetes.

"The data in this study suggest that physical training can be valuable in the treatment of . . . maturity-onset diabetes," concluded Dr. Soman and his colleagues in the *New England Journal of Medicine*.

Shape May Signal Diabetes

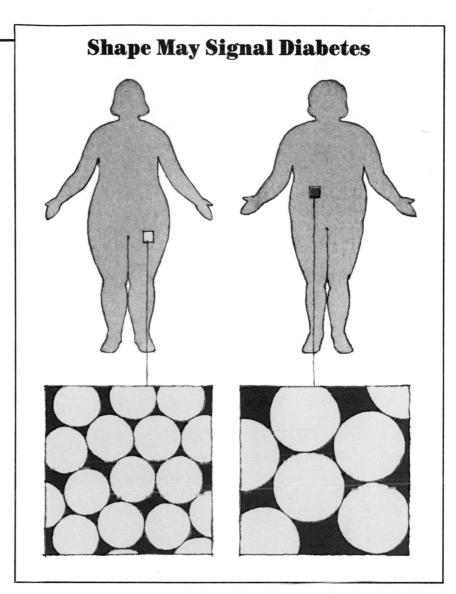

Exercise is important for yet another reason. It helps keep the platelets in the blood from sticking together. Platelets are tiny disk-shaped clotting elements in the blood that are *supposed* to bunch together when you cut yourself. Problems start when they jump the gun, sticking together when there's no cut. In diabetics, that abnormal clotting can cause problems like diabetic retinopathy, tiny hemorrhages in the eyes that can lead to blindness.

Peter Forsham, M.D., at the University of California, San Francisco, studied the effect of exercise on the platelets of six juvenile diabetics. He found that the stickiness of platelets decreased after exercise by 21 percent, and says that exercise may help prevent diabetic retinopathy.

First comes fat and then, if there's enough fat, comes diabetes. But now researchers at the Medical College of Wisconsin are adding a new fold to the story. It seems *where* a woman is fat may be just as important.

Ahmed H. Kissebah, M.D., a professor of medicine who directs the university's clinical research center, conducted a survey of 15,500 women. He found that among the women who carry their extra weight above the waist, 16 percent had diabetes, whereas only 3 percent of those with heavy hips and thighs had diabetes. Check your own figure with those illustrated above.

You'll notice, too, that the woman on the left has smaller fat cells, but lots of them. The woman on the right has fewer but larger cells. These are the type that shape the diabetes-prone body.

8

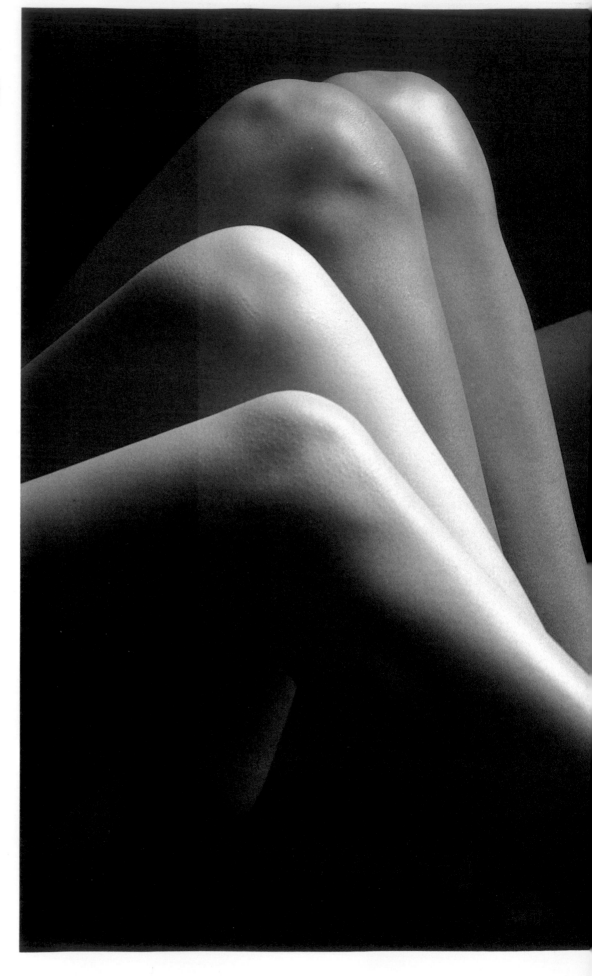

Diet Rules the Skin's Health

What you eat plays a big role in preventing skin diseases like psoriasis, shingles and acne.

The skin is the mirror of a person's inner health. It is often the first indicator of stress, joy or pain. The blood vessels in our face dilate when we're surprised or embarrassed, making it a hot, rose-colored hue. Goose bumps spread over our body when we're cold or frightened. If we're injured the skin puffs up; one of the first questions asked when someone falls is, "Is there any swelling?"

We depend on our skin, but because it is so tolerant of injury and so quick to repair itself, we often take it for granted. That is, until disease strikes. Then we search for cures, wondering why the skin has turned on us. But wouldn't it be better to prevent skin disease in the first place? While some of the diseases described in this chapter are as old as man and twice as stubborn, all of them can be prevented—or at least controlled—with good diet and commonsense self-care. Two of the diseases—shingles and psoriasis—are chronic, meaning they can surface again and again in some people, and can't ever be cured. But to look at them as never-ending problems is self-defeating. Instead, they must be seen as troublemakers only when the symptoms are present. Then, by successfully treating those symptoms, you beat the disease. And the symptoms of most skin diseases *can* be eradicated.

Many of the treatments in this chapter are "natural," which means they aren't going to cause a lot of dangerous side effects, and are usually fairly inexpensive. All of them will make you feel better and your healthy skin will tell people you are fit, comfortable and happy.

When you take care of the skin you are taking care of the body's largest organ. That's right, organ. Just like the heart, liver and kidneys. Though it is difficult to play favorites, the skin is certainly one of the most important organs.

Without it, you'd be a rather disorganized mess. So play it safe and treat your skin right by eating the healthiest foods. If disease does strike, strike back with proper nutrition. Remember, your skin is a reflection of you. Let that image be a healthy one.

PSORIASIS DOESN'T HAVE TO BREAK YOUR HEART

Psoriasis has been known at least since biblical times, and people have been hunting for a cure ever since.

Though "cures" have come and gone, no one has found a way to guarantee freedom from psoriasis. But psoriatic people needn't despair. They should try to accept the fact that their psoriasis is chronic and may return, and then concentrate on treating the symptoms. By following the simple procedures in this section, the disease *can* be controlled.

Psoriasis is characterized by scaly patches that usually first appear on the arms and legs or head. These patches, called plaques, can be limited to one area or spread over the whole body. There is little rhyme or reason to where and how extensive the scales are in any individual.

If the plaques appear, it means your skin cells are multiplying at a rate about seven times faster than normal. Your goal is to slow them down. Chances are you can—with a simple change in diet and exposure to safe amounts of ultraviolet light rays, like those from the sun. Evidence also points to vitamins and minerals as answers to what has become known as "the heartbreak of psoriasis."

COMMON PROTEIN LINKED TO PSORIASIS

French researchers may have found a link between the most common type of psoriasis and problems digesting gluten—a protein found in grains such as wheat, rye, barley and oats. Eleven people with stubborn and severe psoriasis who were also gluten intolerant were put on a gluten-free diet. Eliminating the troublesome grains resulted in "remarkable improvements in these patients and less frequent relapses," said the researchers. They put their results to the ultimate test by reintroducing gluten to the diet of one person whose psoriasis had completely disappeared. It took only three days on the gluten diet for psoriasis to reappear. If you suspect you might be gluten intolerant, try abstaining from gluten-containing grains. Watch your psoriasis. If it disappears, stay off those grains for good and find substitutes such as rice, millet, corn and amaranth, or switch to flours made from nongrain vegetables such as potatoes or soybeans.

A TREATMENT THAT MAKES LIGHT OF PLAQUES

It turns out that one of the best psoriasis treatments may be a vacation!

Ultraviolet light, the kind that comes naturally from the sun, is effective in treating psoriasis. The plaques clear up after long-term exposure to the long waves in ultraviolet light. The problem has always been that sunlight also has short waves, which can burn the skin and lead to serious problems such as cancer. So, while a person who lies out in the backyard for psoriasis sun treatment is doing himself good, he's also risking a sunburn that can aggravate psoriasis.

However, an Israeli resort offers the promise that you can come to life at the Dead Sea. The sea is located south of Jerusalem at 1,300 feet *below* sea level, about six times lower than Death Valley. The sunlight reaching the shore of the Dead Sea passes through a thick atmospheric layer, which acts as a filter, screening out the short, harmful rays of light and letting the long, beneficial rays come through. Guests generally spend four weeks at the spa sunning themselves, swimming in the buoyant, super-salty sea and relaxing as at any other resort.

According to the Israel Society of Dermatology, the spa is a great success, with a majority of visitors improving or recovering completely after spending four weeks at the spa. If plaques recurred, they generally

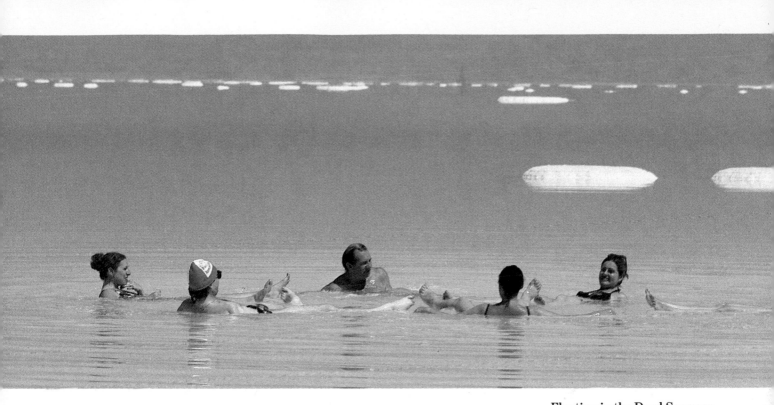

were milder than those that reappeared after more traditional therapies.

HOME TREATMENT

If you can't make it all the way to the Dead Sea, and decide instead to sun yourself in your own backyard, be careful. Jim Stover, M.D., of the Psoriasis Treatment Center of Tulane University in New Orleans recommends that people work up to spending 30 minutes in the sun in the middle of the day. But, he says, "You can bake yourself too much, and the psoriasis will flare up. Don't do it to the point of burning."

Zinc has come to the rescue of the many psoriatics who develop arthritis as a result of their skin disorder. This common sideline symptom of psoriasis—you usually develop psoriasis long before you get psoriatic arthritis—is a painful, crippling complication that aggravates the problems already caused by unsightly plaques. But take heart—and take zinc. Several studies have shown that zinc can provide long-term, safe and inexpensive relief from psoriatic arthritis.

Danish researchers studied the effect zinc had on 24 people who had been suffering with psoriatic arthritis for long periods of time. Half of the patients were given zinc for six weeks and the other half were given a harmless, ineffective placebo. The psoriasis patients who took zinc showed great improvement in their arthritis. The researchers concluded that "oral zinc sulphate seems to be valuable in the treatment of psoriatic arthritis."

Their conclusion is backed up by work done at the University of Glasgow, Scotland, where doctors measured the levels of zinc in 31 hospital patients with psoriasis. They found that this group had significantly lower levels of zinc in their blood than a similar group of nonpsoriatics.

INFANTS PROTECTED BY ZINC

Acrodermatitis enteropathica (AE) is a chilling disease because it most often strikes defenseless infants, making their lives miserable due to the severe skin lesions, diarrhea and hair loss that are typical of the disease. Fortunately, this sometimes lethal condition is simply and easily treated by adding zinc to the diet.

The disease is usually associated with breastfeeding—from the day of birth to the day of weaning. Babies come into the world ready for action. They need nutrients right away and the mother is usually well equipped to supply them. However, some

Floating in the Dead Sea near Jerusalem is easy because the salt-saturated water is extra buoyant. It's also good for psoriasis sufferers because the low-level ultraviolet light from the sun helps heal bothersome skin plaques. And, because the resort is well below sea level, harmful sun rays are filtered out by the atmosphere, reducing the risk of sunburn, which can aggravate psoriasis. People from all over the world spend their vacations at the Dead Sea resorts. Psoriasis sufferers find it comforting to be around other people with the same problem. And everyone enjoys the sand, water and sun.

breastfed babies nevertheless developed AE. For years scientists were puzzled by the quirk: Infants who were deficient in zinc had mothers whose milk should have been adequate. In fact, when the mothers were tested, their bodies had adequate levels of zinc. Why should their babies suffer from a deficiency?

Doctors at the University of Connecticut and the University of Colorado, Denver, studied two infants and found the answer to the puzzle. The doctors' subjects were two breastfed nine-month-old infants who had AE due to zinc deficiencies. Even when the mothers were given oral zinc supplements, the zinc levels in their milk remained low. The doctors concluded from this that breast milk can be zinc deficient because of a defect in mammary secretions, and that this may cause AE. Fortunately, when the infants were given oral zinc supplements, their zinc levels became normal and their AE symptoms disappeared.

STILL OTHER CAUSES

But AE is a complex disease, and deficient mammary secretions don't

completely explain it. For example, AE also may occur when a previously healthy infant is weaned from human milk to cow's milk, even though cow's milk contains more zinc than human milk.

If your child exhibits the rash, hair loss and dry skin of AE *after* he is weaned, check with your doctor and make sure the baby is given zinc. It seems there is an inherited disorder that leaves infants with very low levels of an acid necessary to break down zinc. Human milk contains much more of this acid than cow's milk—a case of Mother Nature providing natural relief for the disease.

If there is a history of AE in your family, make sure that your doctor knows about it so your infant can be checked for this inherited disorder. If there is a potential problem, zinc supplements can help avert it.

Occasionally adults and older children can develop AE, especially if they are receiving total parenteral nutrition (TPN)—a liquid nutrient given intravenously to people with severe digestive problems and to other hospital patients. The solutions sometimes are deficient in zinc. If you (or anyone in your family) is given TPN for any length of time, check with the doctor to be certain you are receiving enough zinc.

SHORT-CIRCUITING SHINGLES

If you had chicken pox when you were a child, you are a candidate for shingles. But don't start worrying. While 90 percent of the population has had chicken pox and therefore carries the virus that can eventually erupt in shingles, only 10 percent ever will be afflicted. Those that do suffer the pain should know that there is a variety of safe, natural remedies that may help alleviate the suffering or prevent it from ever occurring again.

Shingles is the common name for herpes zoster, part of a family of viruses that includes genital herpes, cold sores, mononucleosis and chicken pox. The viruses are all related, but only chicken pox seems to have close

Looking at your skin, you see a fairly smooth surface, perhaps punctuated by hairs, moles and a few wrinkles. But that is only the surface layer. The skin is deeper than you may think. Underneath the outer layer is a complex group of blood vessels, fat cells and glands which allow the body to perspire and feel pain, and which otherwise work to keep the body together and functioning well. Healthy skin means more than outward appearance. Taking care of the inside layers is important, too.

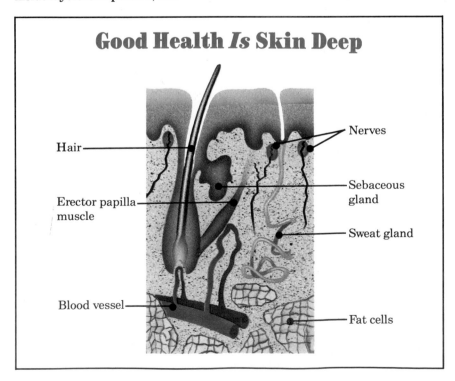

Good Health *Is* Skin Deep

Hair

Erector papilla muscle

Blood vessel

Nerves

Sebaceous gland

Sweat gland

Fat cells

ties to shingles. The chicken pox virus will retreat into the nerve ganglia as the childhood disease subsides and will usually remain peacefully in the body for life. Unfortunately, the virus sometimes pops back to life—usually in people who are over 50 years old—and causes shingles. The attack begins with pain under the skin, fever or a headache. After several days, a rash of fluid-filled blisters appears, usually on one side of the trunk or face. Pain, often strong enough to drive a person to despair, usually accompanies the rash. If you have shingles, you can keep suffering to a minimum by employing several simple methods of treating the symptoms.

The first step is to relieve any discomfort the shingles eruption might be causing. Richard T. Johnson, M.D., professor of microbiology and neuroscience at Johns Hopkins University School of Medicine in Baltimore, advises patients to put talcum powder or calamine lotion on the rash. Experience has taught Dr. Johnson that young shingles sufferers—those few who develop the condition before they reach middle age—usually experience only a mild eruption and only mild discomfort.

If simple lotions don't take care of your problem, try vitamins.

RELIEF WITH VITAMIN C

Numerous reports have shown dramatic relief from shingles after taking large amounts of vitamin C. J. N. Dizon, M.D., of New York City, wrote to *Skin and Allergy News,* saying that he has great success treating shingles patients with 10 grams of vitamin C daily (a level of intake that should be used only under a doctor's supervision). The lesions usually dry up within two to five days. "I told another physician of these findings," says Dr. Dizon. "When he tried the same on his patients, he had similar results."

A North Carolina doctor also reported success with vitamin C. Frederick Klenner, M.D., treated eight shingles patients with injections of 2 to 3 grams of vitamin C every 12 hours and 1 gram orally

every 2 hours. All but one of the subjects experienced substantial relief within 72 hours. (Again, take this much C only under a doctor's care.)

RELIEF FROM LONG-TERM PAIN

Vitamins also are used to treat shingles pain—including the tormenting, demoralizing generalized pain that sometimes lasts for years after the lesions disappear, causing

Ichthyosis

Ichthyosis – ich-thy-o-sis/ikthē′ ō-sės/ n, pl ichthyo ses/-ō, sēz/ [NL, fr. ichthy- + -osis]: a congenital disease usu. of hereditary origin characterized by skin that is rough, thick and scaly and resembles that of a fish—called also fishskin disease.

Ichthyosis. It's an unusual name, but a fairly common disease, affecting 1 in 250 Americans. The disease results in peeling, sometimes so severe that ichthyosis victims can become social cripples because of their disfigurement. Fortunately, most cases are mild.

Ichthyosis usually appears only as dry skin—the victims of this inherited disease may not even know they have it. One California dermatologist, working at the Veterans' Administration Hospital and the University of California in San Francisco, says that people with mild cases of dry, flaky ichthyosis don't need to see a doctor. For them, home treatment is usually effective. First, sufferers should avoid cold, dry weather. For those who live in intemperate climates, a good heater and humidifier will help. In addition, topical lubricants can usually relieve mild cases of ichthyosis. Try adding bath oil to the water when you bathe, or apply a cream directly to the affected area.

Finally, ichthyosis always first appears during childhood. If it crops up in an adult, it may be a sign of more serious problems, even cancer, so see a doctor.

many people to just give up.

Such discomfort often isn't necessary, according to John G. McConahy, M.D., a dermatologist practicing in New Castle, Pennsylvania. He routinely gives his shingles patients vitamins C and B complex and a multivitamin and mineral tablet along with corticosteroids.

"For best results," Dr. McConahy says, "treatment should be started as soon as the sores appear and then continued for two weeks. With that regimen, I've never had a patient whose pain lasted longer than six weeks. The fact is, 70 percent of the pain is gone within two weeks after the sores have disappeared."

Dr. McConahy thinks that vitamins C and B complex help the nerve cells regenerate and rebuild. "The substance that surrounds the nerve fibers (called the sheath) is derived from these very same vitamins."

Vitamin E also seems to help relieve the sometimes excruciating long-term shingles pain. Richard Mihan, M.D., of the University of Southern California School of Medicine, and Samuel Ayres, M.D., have effectively helped many long-term pain sufferers with it.

The two doctors treated a group of 13 people who had experienced chronic pain from shingles. During four years' time they were given both oral doses of vitamin E (400 to 1,600 I.U. daily) and a cream applied directly to the sores each day.

Eleven of the patients had suffered from moderate to severe pain for over six months. Seven of those had suffered for over 1 year; 1 had been in pain for 13 years and another for 19 years! The vitamin helped nine of the patients, including the two long-term shingles sufferers. All nine experienced almost total relief from their pain. The remaining four patients, while not as lucky as the rest, did show some improvement, too. (Any intake of vitamin E over 800 I.U. a day should be subject to your doctor's approval.)

"The mechanism by which vitamin E relieves the persistent pain of post-herpes zoster neuralgia is not known," concluded Dr. Mihan and Dr. Ayres, "but in view of its long duration in many of our cases, we do not believe it is coincidence. Vitamin E may not be 100 percent effective, but many of our patients get relief from persistent pain."

The Black and White of Skin Disease

Dermatologists in the United States are trained to treat light-colored, Caucasian skin. But blacks have skin problems, too, and many people aren't aware that darker skin sometimes reacts differently to a "standard" treatment. For example, certain drugs that have no adverse effects on light skin can cause light or dark spots on black skin. One such drug is the peeling agent used for acne treatments, which may leave the skin noticeably darker than it was before. Freezing is a common way to rid a patient of warts. But when black skin is frozen, it can result in loss of pigment for an area 3 times the size of the wart. By far the most common dermatological problem in black men results from shaving. The curly facial hair, shortened by the razor, turns back toward the skin, becomes ingrown and can cause sores. The treatment is to let the hair grow for several weeks until the natural tension causes the ingrown ends of the hairs to pop out of the skin.

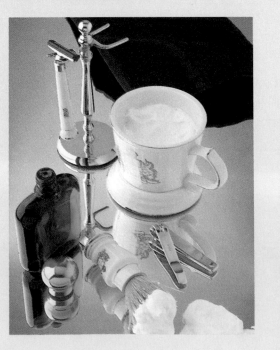

ABOLISH ADULT ACNE

Almost everyone gets acne at one time or another. There is just no way around it. Acne is usually just a minor blemish on the surface of your life, the kind of health problem that does nothing more serious than make you nervous before the Senior Prom. However, some people carry their acne into adulthood, and then it's no laughing matter. This severe form of acne is a real troublemaker that leaves not only ugly physical scars on the face but also emotional scars which sometimes last for life.

Despite the large number of people disfigured by cystic acne, medical science has yet to find a cure. Yet, there is strong evidence that a nutritional approach to treating this disease may be the "hidden" answer that doctors have spent years hunting. And once again, the solution is zinc.

Dermatologists (specialists in skin disorders) have long advocated *eliminating* certain foods like chocolate from the diet. However, it turns out that chocolate, nuts and other traditional "no-no's" have little bearing on the development or continuance of acne. Only recently has the medical establishment discovered a straighter, truer path, realizing that *adding* certain foods—specifically those rich in zinc—is the way to treat acne.

Researchers have shown that a low-zinc diet will aggravate a case of acne in as few as 10 to 14 days. This inflammation may result simply because the outer layer of the skin "requires five to six times as much zinc as the dermis (underlying layer)," says Kenneth H. Neldner, M.D., a dermatologist in Denver.

ZINC VS. ANTIBIOTICS

The antibiotic tetracycline has been the primary agent used in the past by dermatologists to protect this layer of skin. But a Swedish study has shown that zinc is at least as effective—and zinc doesn't have the side effects that tetracycline does, like intestinal upset and lowered immunity. Gerd Michaëlsson, M.D., of Uppsala, Sweden, ran a comparison test. He gave 19 acne patients

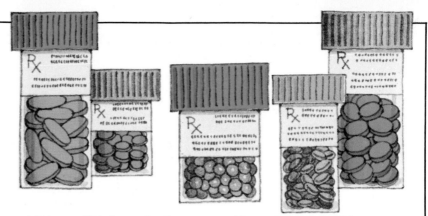

Your Skin: A Target for Side Effects

We commonly enlist various drugs to help us wage war on headaches, pneumonia, ulcers, sore throats and upset stomachs. Frequent unwanted by-products of these battles for health include decidedly unhealthy skin conditions such as measleslike rashes, inflamed pimples, scales and discolored spots. Skin eruptions are the most frequent adverse reaction to drugs—more common than nausea, drowsiness and nervousness.

Prescribed drugs like corticosteroids, lithium and bromides cause pimples, as do over-the-counter vitamins and minerals containing iodides.

Antibiotics like penicillin and tetracycline and depressants like barbiturates and thiazides (Valium) sometimes lead to a rash that resembles measles or scarlet fever. Barbiturates, codeine, insulin, penicillin and even aspirin can cause red, itchy hives. Oral contraceptives can lead to serious blisters on the skin and in the mouth and yellowish-brown patches on the forehead and cheeks.

These reactions can occur suddenly, even in someone who has safely taken the drug for years. If you suspect trouble, see your doctor about a substitute drug. Or better yet, find a natural treatment.

135 milligrams of zinc a day and started a second group of 18 on 750 milligrams a day of tetracycline. After 12 weeks, both groups averaged a 67 percent improvement in their complexions.

Still other Swedish dermatologists conducted a study of 91 patients with moderately severe acne. Zinc was given to 48, while the remaining 43 received a placebo. According to the researchers, "significantly better results were demonstrated in favor of zinc after 12 weeks."

Zinc may help clear acne in several ways: by reducing irritation and inflammation; by helping damaged skin to heal quickly; or by helping the liver release vitamin A in the body. This vitamin, which is also known to have an anti-inflammatory effect, has been touted since the mid-1970s as a good treatment for severe adult acne, especially when combined with vitamin E.

The duo seems to work well because vitamin E has a synergistic, or boosting, effect on vitamin A. In one experiment, over 100 patients were treated with daily doses of 100,000 I.U. of vitamin A and 800 I.U. of vitamin E. Within a matter of weeks, most of the patients responded well to the therapy, and thereafter were able to keep their skin clear with regular lower doses of the vitamins. (Large doses of vitamin A—anything over 25,000 I.U. daily—should only be taken with your doctor's okay.)

Fallout from Acne Therapy

Both sunlamps and X rays were used to treat people with severe acne, but they fell from grace in the late 1970s. The reason: The treatments may contribute to cancer. Sunlamps went dark because of the connection between ultraviolet light and skin cancer. X ray treatments have been linked with cancer of the thyroid and breast.

Douglas B. Thomson, M.D., working at the Geisinger Medical Center, Danville, Pennsylvania, studied a group of 296 patients who had received radiation for their acne. Surprisingly (and frighteningly), two thyroid cancers were discovered. Dr. Thomson recommends that people who were given radiation therapy for acne have yearly thyroid checkups.

Norman Simon, M.D., of the Mt. Sinai School of Medicine, New York, studied 16 women with breast cancer who had been treated with radiation for acne in their youth. He concluded that "the radiation contributed causally to the breast cancers," and suggests that women who have been irradiated be especially watchful for signs of breast cancer.

FIBER FIGHTS ACNE

Replacing the fats in your diet with some high-fiber foods like bran, sweet potatoes and blackberries might help clear up acne, according to a Maryland doctor.

William H. Kaufman, M.D., reported in the *Archives of Dermatology* that he had "several highly motivated patients with acne who had a rapid, indeed almost abrupt, clearing of their skin through correction of faulty bowel elimination by means of a daily serving of about 1 ounce of an all-bran breakfast cereal.

"I believe correction of constipation is a favorable influence on acne," Dr. Kaufman wrote. Though no clinical studies back up Dr. Kaufman's belief, the success of his patients suggests that fiber may be just what acne sufferers need.

BEDSORES CAN BE HEALED

Bedsores. They afflict millions of Americans every year, especially those who are old or paraplegic. Often institutionalized, and almost always bedridden, these people are the most frequent victims of bedsores. But there is no reason for these painful lesions to be a fact of life. Good care and nutrition can usually prevent them.

The medical term for bedsores is decubitis ulcers, from the Latin word for lying down, because the sores strike people who are unable to move for long periods of time. The body's weight on pressure points such as elbows and hips closes tiny blood vessels that normally give the skin and flesh nourishment. The deprived tissue can eventually become ulcerous. But if the pressure is relieved occasionally and the body has a good supply of nutrients to send to the skin, the chance of developing bedsores is greatly reduced.

One of the most important tissue-fortifying vitamins is vitamin C, which helps build collagen, a protein vitally involved in tissue repair.

T. V. Taylor, M.D., of the University Hospital of South Manchester,

England, gave ten bedsore patients 500 milligrams of vitamin C twice daily and ten others a placebo twice a day. One month after the experiment began, the placebo group had only a 42 percent reduction in the size of their sores. But the group that took the real vitamin C showed an 84 percent reduction in bedsore size.

ZINC TO THE RESCUE

After the surface of the skin has been breached by an injury or a wound such as a bedsore, the body sets up a two-pronged emergency relief program. First, zinc is rushed from other areas to the wound site, where the mineral helps build collagen and fight infections. Second, to protect damaged tissues that are especially vulnerable to attack by harmful bacteria and viruses, zinc boosts the power of the immune system's cells, which circulate throughout the body in the blood.

Zinc can't be stored in great amounts in our bodies, so it is important to take supplements when bedsores are present. The RDA is 15 milligrams for healthy adults, but many scientists believe the RDA is too low, especially for those over 50 years old.

Yet, even with sufficient zinc, bedsores will occur unless certain commonsense precautions are taken. A person at risk should be turned in bed every two hours to relieve pressure; the pressure points should be checked every eight hours for injury; the skin should be kept clean with gentle soap and water; and if the skin is dry, petroleum jelly should be applied.

In addition, certain types of beds will help relieve excess pressure on the skin and allow air to circulate freely. Water beds cushion the body and help relieve pressure. (And Medicare will pick up the tab.) There are also "egg crate" mattresses— mattresses that look just like egg cartons, with hills and valleys made of foam—that reduce the area of pressure and also allow air to circulate under the body. Perhaps the most unusual bed is a tank filled with about 1,500 pounds of glass beads—

finer than sand—that are blown around the back of the patient to make a perfect air-filled cushion.

HOW TO TREAT ACTIVE SORES

If, after taking these preventive measures, bedsores still form, there are a few steps that can be taken to hasten healing. One of the best is reaching for the sugar bowl. James W. Barnes, Jr., M.D., of Bowie, Maryland, claims a healing rate of close to 80 percent when he packs the ulcers with a mixture of finely ground white sugar and other substances and wraps the wounds in airtight dressings.

Why sugar? Because it has several special properties. Its acidity increases dilation of the blood vessels, drawing more healing agents to the sore. The sucrose kills bacteria and the granules gently irritate the sore, stimulating repair.

Physicians also apply nutrient solutions directly to the wounds to supplement nutrients already working from within the body. Anthony N. Silvetti, M.D., of Bethany Methodist Hospital in Chicago, has had at least partial success with all but 3 percent of 500 patients using a combination of carbohydrates, amino acids and vitamin C.

While Dr. Silvetti's success is encouraging, don't wait for bedsores to strike before taking positive action. Prevent them in the first place by providing the invalid with proper nutrition and good care.

Bees Beat Bedsores

One of the newest natural buzzwords in medicine is honey. The very honey you drizzle into your tea can effectively heal many wounds and infections— including bedsores—according to physicians at the Barrhead Hospital in Alberta, Canada, as reported in the prestigious British journal *Lancet*.

Honey is either spread on gauze or packed directly into the sore, which is then wrapped tightly and left to heal. It works well as an antibiotic because it "creates an instant unfavorable environment for bacterial growth," say the doctors. And no bacteria means no infection. Unlike antibiotics, honey is inexpensive, effective and natural.

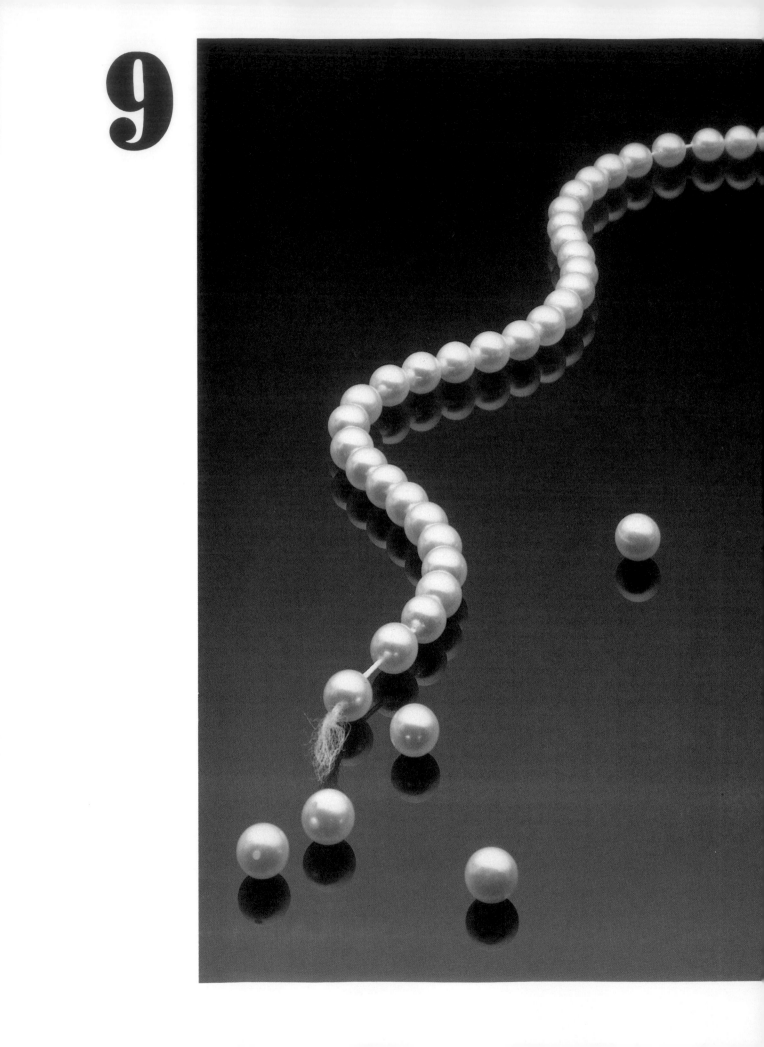

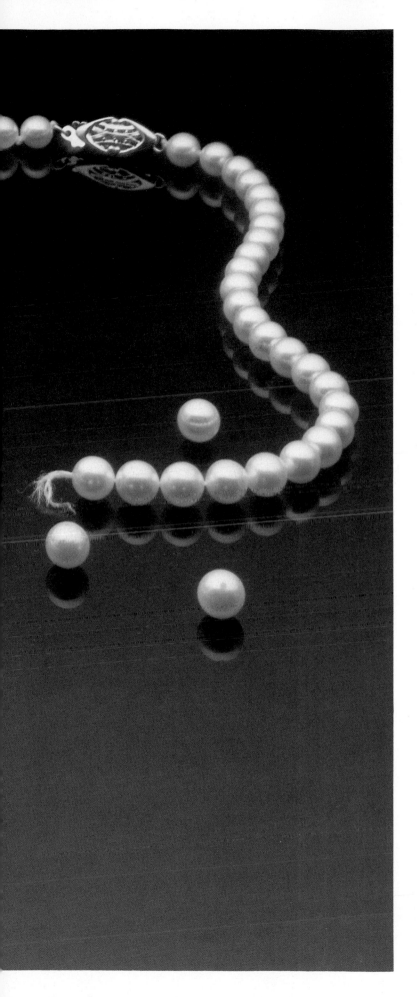

Caring for the Health of Women

Prevention and knowledge have revolutionized women's health care.

The movement is marked not by marches, placards and speeches but by quieter sounds—the rustling of pages, soft words of advice and comfort, subtle lifestyle changes and more open communication. Nonetheless, women's health care is being revolutionized, slowly but steadily evolving so that now women are becoming equal partners in their own medical destinies.

Women are learning to apply the ultimate "right to know" standard to their own bodies in order to become educated medical consumers. This especially applies to women's reproductive health, an area that has finally, over the past decade, received serious medical attention. With this heightened concern has come an increased emphasis on self-care and natural remedies. For centuries, long before there were doctors, hospitals and obstetrical units, women had to depend on instinct and folk wisdom. Thus, a return to self-care treatments and preventive medicine, emphasizing diet, exercise and similar positive steps, is all the more natural.

Unlike past centuries, however, when frank discussion of women's health problems and even certain terms were taboo, such issues have come out into the open. For the first time, serious attention has been paid to premenstrual syndrome (PMS) and how women can learn to control it through changes in diet and lifestyle. Women are learning more about the role of vitamins in overcoming menstrual difficulties such as heavy bleeding and cramps. Other disorders now receiving closer medical study include pelvic inflammatory disease (PID), an infection that may lead to infertility if it goes unchecked, and endometriosis, a painful disorder of the uterine lining. Infertile couples are also finding ways to reverse their problems through natural treatments. The key to remaining healthy is actively applied self-knowledge. With this key, women are becoming equal partners in the medical system.

PREVENTING PMS

Looking at the door, which was splintered and full of huge nicks, Carol felt sure that she could not have been the one who damaged it. But the bruises on her hands said differently. The night before, Carol had been arguing with her boyfriend when she lost control of her anger and began striking the bedroom door with her fists and then bashing it with an umbrella. Such outbursts seemed to happen every few weeks, visiting her like unwelcome strangers.

When Carol asked her doctor about these violent episodes, the first words out of his mouth were, "Go to a psychiatrist." When therapy did not help, Carol's doctor prescribed tranquilizers, but they only made her feel worse.

Carol's experience with PMS is all too common. An estimated 70 to 90 percent of women suffer some form of this troubling problem, which is marked by symptoms that may occur at any time between ovulation and the menstrual period.

Whether or not PMS has psychological components, its symptoms have been linked to hormonal and other physical causes as well. Women need not feel that premenstrual distress is the result of a hypersensitive imagination or psychological weakness of any sort. The first step is to make sure your problems are in fact related to your menstrual cycle and not to some other problem. The best way to do this is to chart your symptoms.

At the PMS Medical Group in New York City, a private clinic begun by Joseph Martorano, M.D., patients are instructed to keep a daily log of their mood (rating it from 1 to 10) and any symptoms, such as depression or headaches. They also record their weight, to gauge water retention, and basal body temperature, to determine the time of ovulation. In a separate notebook, the women keep a daily log of what they eat and the vitamin and mineral supplements they take. Using this information,

the medical center staff can devise certain steps to avert PMS.

The solution is not necessarily in a pill bottle. Instead, a more holistic, natural approach can beat PMS, especially by combating the two major causes of the troubling symptoms—a hormone imbalance and hypoglycemia (low blood sugar).

Hypoglycemia is believed to be at the core of many premenstrual problems, such as fatigue and anxiety. Blood sugar denotes the amount of glucose—the only source of food for the brain and most body cells—in the blood. If there is a low level of glucose, the brain and other body cells are, in effect, starved and cannot function properly.

Research also indicates that a shortage of progesterone, the hormone that, among other things, keeps water from accumulating in the body, may spur many PMS symptoms. Even worse, says Dr. Martorano, is the effect of inadequate levels of progesterone on sugar metabolism. Without this hormone, the body fails to convert sugar properly, which results in symptoms that accompany hypoglycemia, including headaches, faintness and panic attacks, among other problems.

The exact steps you can take to control PMS depend on your symptoms, but here are some tips.

Cut Down Your Intake of Sodium and Stay Away from Refined Sugar. Salt is a prime culprit in the body's retention of fluid. Season food with lemon and herbs, remove salt shakers from the table and determine the hidden sources of salt in your diet, such as canned foods. Refined sugars, which are simple carbohydrates, enter the bloodstream quickly, provoking a sudden spurt of insulin that can knock your blood sugar down to fasting level.

Eat Complex Carbohydrates and High-Protein Foods. These include whole grain breads, fresh fruits, lean meats and steamed or raw vegetables. Besides being packed with nutrients, these foods, which are broken down more gradually than simple carbohydrates, assure the bloodstream a constant glucose supply.

The Dos and Don'ts of Cramps

1. **Do** exercise to relax and ease the pain.
2. **Do** get plenty of calcium daily (800 to 1,000 milligrams).
3. **Do** drink herbal tea or sit in a hot tub. Heat soothes pain.
4. **Don't** drink coffee, tea or alcohol.
5. **Don't** go on birth control pills to ease cramps. The risks aren't worth it.
6. **Do** take heart. Cramps often lessen with age.

Lean Bodies and Late Menstruation—A Connection

When girls fail to begin menstruation by a normal age (usually before the age of 16), the condition—which is not necessarily a health problem—is known as amenorrhea. One factor believed to have a big impact on the start of menstruation is athletic training. Allan J. Ryan, M.D., calls intense athletic training probably "the most common cause of delayed menarche in this country today." Runners and gymnasts who are extremely thin have been found to experience delayed onset of their periods, and ballet dancers also often begin menstruating later in life. In fact, dancers and athletes often do not begin to menstruate until after they quit intense training.

One plausible reason is the effect of body fat on hormone levels. Fat plays a key role in the release of estrogen. Several researchers, including R. E. Frisch, Ph.D., say a woman must maintain a specific percentage of body fat—believed to be at least 17 percent—in order for estrogen production to regulate the menstrual cycle. Those who stay lean because of intense training may find that their body's fat composition dips below the necessary threshold for hormone regulation. A study of 21 Harvard swimmers and 17 runners found that each year of training before menstruation delayed the onset of periods by an average of 5 months. But researchers also found that stopping training, reducing its intensity or ensuring good nutrition enables menstruation to proceed normally.

Eat Smaller, More Frequent Meals. At the PMS Medical Group, patients are told to eat six medium-size meals and three mini-meals or snacks to help stabilize the body's conversion of food to glucose.

Cut Out Caffeine and Alcohol. Caffeine has been known to intensify PMS symptoms such as irritability and breast tenderness. By drinking alcohol, you infuse the bloodstream with loads of carbohydrates.

Use a Sound Vitamin and Mineral Supplement Program. Research has shown that certain nutrient deficiencies can trigger PMS symptoms. The PMS Medical Group advises the following daily program: one stress formula multivitamin and mineral tablet; one 50-milligram B_6 tablet; one 100-milligram timed-release B complex vitamin tablet; 500 milligrams of evening primrose oil taken in six doses; and 100 micrograms of chromium.

Exercise Regularly. Both aerobic and relaxation exercises can upgrade your overall fitness, making you less vulnerable to stress.

This program has been found to be effective for 70 percent of the PMS Medical Group patients. The remainder are given natural progesterone on a six-month trial basis.

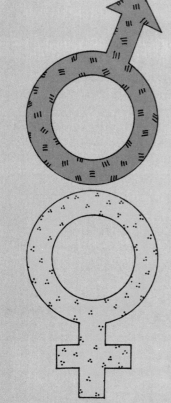

Toxic-Shock Syndrome—It's Not for Women Only

Toxic-shock syndrome has come to be associated with women and menstrual periods to the extent that some call it the "tampon disease." It's no wonder, since publicity about the potentially fatal illness, which surged in mid-1980, linked TSS to tampons. You're mistaken, however, if you think women are the only ones who can get toxic-shock syndrome. Men have gotten TSS also. In a review of 54 cases of TSS occurring over a 5-year period, researchers at the Centers for Disease Control in Atlanta reported that 17 males had contracted the disease. In one instance, a 14-year-old boy developed toxic-shock syndrome when a foot injury, sustained while riding his bicycle, became infected. Doctors found that the bacterium *Staphylococcus aureus,* which is believed to produce the toxin in TSS, was present in the boy's wound. While the majority of TSS victims are menstruating women, researchers point out that the proportion of cases unrelated to menstruation has increased. TSS can befall anyone with any type of staphylococcal infection, occurring in surgical incisions, burns or insect bites. The early symptoms are the same for both males and females: rash, fever, diarrhea and vomiting.

CURING CRAMPS

Nearly half of all young women suffer menstrual cramps, but, thankfully, these spasmodic uterine pains usually grow milder as women mature.

Cramps fall into two categories: primary dysmenorrhea and secondary dysmenorrhea. The primary type is the pain that typically strikes when the menstrual flow begins. It does not signify serious disorder. Secondary dysmenorrhea, or severe cramping, usually indicates a serious problem, such as fibroid tumors, pelvic inflammatory disease or endometriosis.

As with PMS, there are nondrug alternatives to battling cramps. Exercise, especially vigorous daily workouts like jogging, swimming or aerobic dance, can help prevent cramps in the first place. One study found that eight weeks of bent-knee sit-ups, done daily, meant much less painful periods for 36 college women. (If you try this exercise, start with as many sit-ups as you can do comfortably and increase them gradually.) Vigorous exercise also stimulates the brain and pituitary gland to release natural painkilling substances known as endorphins.

Cramps are believed to be caused by prostaglandins, hormonelike substances that can prompt muscle contraction. Studies have shown that women who suffer from cramps have higher levels of prostaglandins in their menstrual blood than others.

G. E. Desaulniers, M.D., medical director of the Shute Institute in London, Ontario, has found vitamin E to be effective in lessening the intensity of cramps. The vitamin acts as a mild prostaglandin inhibitor and also soothes inflammation and promotes circulation. Dr. Desaulniers recommends dosages of 400 I.U. daily. "We think it's a safer treatment than many others," he says.

TOXIC-SHOCK SYNDROME STILL A THREAT

In 1979, Janice, a 20-year-old college student, had never heard the word "desquamation." Over the next three

Hysterectomy: Too Often Unnecessary

When gynecologists advise women to have hysterectomies, perhaps the doctors should hand them tiny cards that state: "Warning! Hysterectomies may be unnecessary for your health." Many doctors and consumer research groups assert that this operation is being performed far too indiscriminately and exhibits the worst of sexism in medical practices. In his book *Male Practice: How Doctors Manipulate Women*, Robert S. Mendelsohn, M.D., speculates that only about 1 in 5 hysterectomies is justified as a life-saving measure. With 690,000 hysterectomies performed in 1979, Dr. Mendelsohn says this means that some 500,000 women per year are having an unnecessary operation that does not justify the risks. Some hysterectomies are quite justifiable, such as removal of the uterus because of painful fibroid tumors. In other cases, removal of the uterus to prevent cancer makes little sense, considering there is less chance a woman will die from uterine cancer than that she will die from complications due to the hysterectomy. Dr. Mendelsohn asserts that in far too many cases, patients are not being given enough information to make a rational choice. If you're faced with this decision and you're unsure about what to do, seek a second doctor's opinion and carefully weigh all the options.

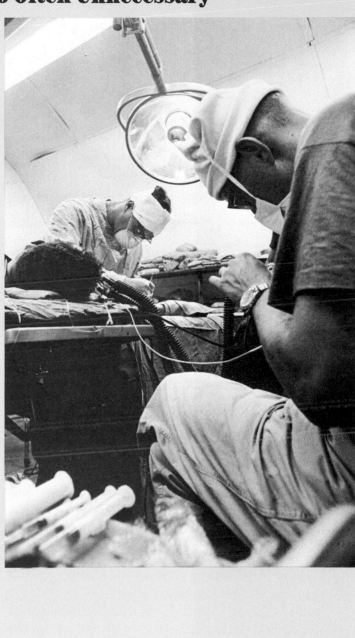

years she would discover its meaning in a very painful way.

The term denotes a peeling or scaling condition, and doctors used it repeatedly to describe the symptom of a mysterious illness that made the skin on Janice's hands and feet peel in layers. Some two years and dozens of doctors later—after she had experienced 13 flare-ups accompanied by a searing rash, fever and headaches— Janice's problem was diagnosed as toxic-shock syndrome (TSS). During this two-year period she had to withdraw from college three times.

Janice was one of 2,297 cases of this potentially fatal disease, which primarily strikes women of childbearing age. As of September 1983, there had been 105 known deaths. Nearly nine out of ten times, women were struck during menstruation, prompting symptoms which include fever, vomiting, diarrhea, headache and rash. At its worst, TSS sends the victim into shock or can bring about respiratory problems or kidney failure. Treatment consists of antibiotics and, in severe cases, hospitalization.

TSS develops when the bacterium *Staphylococcus aureus,* commonly present in the body, produces

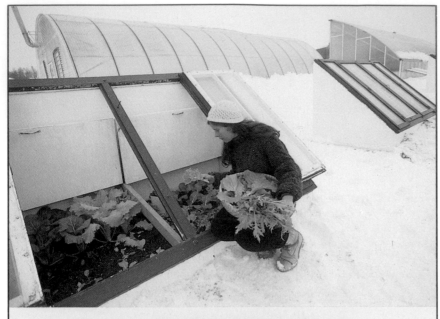

Going the Nutrition Route to Curb Cervical Abnormalities

Eating your broccoli, leaf lettuce and carrots will do far more than just make you slim and healthy. Doctors are finding that good nutrition—and vitamins such as A, C and folate—play an important role in whether a woman has cervical dysplasia, an alteration of cells that's sometimes associated with an early stage of cervical cancer. In a study of 169 women at Albert Einstein College of Medicine, Bronx, N.Y., doctors found that 29 percent of the women who had cervical dysplasia got less than half the Recommended Dietary Allowance of vitamin C daily, compared with only 3 percent in the group who did not have the condition. Other research efforts have shown that dosages of certain vitamins can halt or reverse the cell abnormalities. C. E. Butterworth, M.D., treated oral contraceptive users who had cervical dysplasia with folate supplements and reported significant improvement. In 4 women, the dysplasia regressed to normal. In another experiment, Frank Meyskens, M.D., and Earl Surwit, M.D., treated 21 female patients with a synthetic derivative of vitamin A and got encouraging results. One-quarter of the women had a definite reduction of abnormal cells. Dr. Meyskens is now looking more closely at the effects of vitamin A on cervical dysplasia.

a toxic substance that poisons the system. In 1980 researchers linked toxic shock to the use of tampons.

Although the initial wave of publicity about TSS has subsided, the disease still occurs, striking even nonmenstruating victims. Cases of TSS have been reported in people with infected burns, insect bites and surgical wounds, as well as some diaphragm users.

TSS mainly strikes young menstruating women between the ages of 15 and 19. However, because of the link between tampons and TSS it is clearly advisable for all women to avoid using tampons and switch to sanitary pads whenever feasible. Women who have just given birth should not wear tampons of any kind until the vagina is completely healed.

DRUBBING DUB

For some women, menstrual periods arrive as regularly as the monthly utility bills. Yet for others, periods can sometimes become erratic, a condition known as dysfunctional uterine bleeding, or DUB. This problem frequently occurs in women between the ages of 30 and 50. A woman might find that after years of having clockwork-regular periods she suddenly misses one, then gets a heavy period, spots for 15 days and then has another period six weeks later.

Often, women with DUB are undergoing some stress in their lives, whether physical, such as illness or extreme weight gain, or mental. Such stresses affect the hypothalamus, which regulates the hormone production of the pituitary gland and thus, the menstrual cycle. Carol Jessop, M.D., a California internist who specializes in women's health, attributes many menstrual irregularities to "the 20th-century lifestyle." Often "women with menstrual irregularities don't have time for themselves and don't exercise enough," says Dr. Jessop. Frequently, they are eating on the run, or eating many processed foods and lots of sugar and chocolate.

One good way to know if you are experiencing menstrual irregularities is to keep a calendar of your cycle. If you notice any irregularity—like spotting or heavier periods—watch it closely for a month or two. If periods continue veering from your normal cycle, see a doctor.

Reducing stress, eating well, exercising more and taking adequate vitamin supplements all can get your periods back to normal, says Dr. Jessop. "I tell patients to exercise for 20 minutes at least four times a week—do something aerobic," she explains.

The term DUB is also used to designate failure to ovulate. To determine whether you are ovulating, check your basal body temperature daily (first thing in the morning), using an oral thermometer. The temperature should be about the same until around the thirteenth and fourteenth days of the cycle. During ovulation, it will rise about 2 degrees. A woman with DUB will not experience this temperature increase. If you find this is the case, see your doctor.

THE INFECTION CALLED PID

Mary was "pretty sure" at age 22 that she did not want to have any more children. But, as she recalls, "I didn't want anything permanently done, like sterilization, and I didn't want to take any chances with the Pill."

She was fitted then with an IUD, the intrauterine device that prevents a fertilized egg from implanting in the uterus. After about seven years of using the IUD, Mary began suffering a steady, constant ache, even during intercourse. Her doctor told her she had an infection known as pelvic inflammatory disease that had spread through her fallopian tubes, uterus and ovaries. When antibiotics did not help Mary, her doctor and three specialists told her they wanted to operate to "take a look." Sadly, they did far more, removing Mary's uterus, fallopian tubes and ovaries.

Mary's case is hardly isolated. While the majority of cases of pelvic inflammatory disease stem from sexually transmitted disease or infections associated with surgery or abortion, IUD users are also at increased risk of contracting the infection. An estimated 50,000 IUD users are hospitalized with the disorder each year, and PID is considered the major risk associated with the use of the IUD. Some 200,000 women contract milder forms of the infection each year.

The rate of risk for PID typically ranges from 2 to 20 out of every 100 women per year, but use of the IUD has ballooned that figure at least fourfold. And if you're a young woman, aged 16 to 19, your risk of infection and possible infertility is ten times higher than for women aged 30 to 49, one British study showed.

PID symptoms can either scream their arrival or remain perfectly silent. They include increased menstrual pain and cramps, possibly a bloody or puslike vaginal discharge, painful intercourse, fever, chills or painful urination. Painful cramping is a common side effect of the IUD, but if it is continuous and lasts longer than 24 hours, seek medical attention at once.

Many studies have confirmed that use of the IUD increases the risk of infection, but one study, based on 155 PID sufferers and done over a five-year period, went even further, finding that the Dalkon Shield was even more harmful than the others. In an editorial accompanying the study in the *Journal of the American Medical Association*, Peter Layde, M.D., advised women who use this type of IUD to replace it with another or consider an alternate birth control method.

Early detection of PID is critical, since antibiotics can hold the disease in check and keep it from spreading to the ovaries, fallopian tubes and other parts of the pelvis. At later stages, hospitalization may be required. In the worst cases, scar tissue can block the tubes and cause infertility. Also, if an IUD has prompted heavy bleeding, be sure to take an iron supplement daily to prevent anemia.

Some women may still opt for the IUD despite the risks. Before an IUD is inserted, the doctor should perform an internal exam and a Pap smear. The greatest risk of PID occurs in the first month after IUD insertion but the possibility of

The Problem with Hygiene Products

Many women fail to realize that the vagina has a natural ability to cleanse itself and that feminine hygiene products—douches, deodorant tampons, deodorant sprays and the like—are often far more harmful than hygienic. Two doctors, Hans Neumann, M.D., and Alan DeCherney, M.D., reported in the *New England Journal of Medicine* that 90 percent of the women they treated for pelvic inflammatory disease used vigorous douches. A kindred culprit is feminine hygiene spray, which contains chemicals that can cause irritation and inflammation in vaginal and vulvar tissues. Introducing chemicals into the vagina increases the chances of infection.

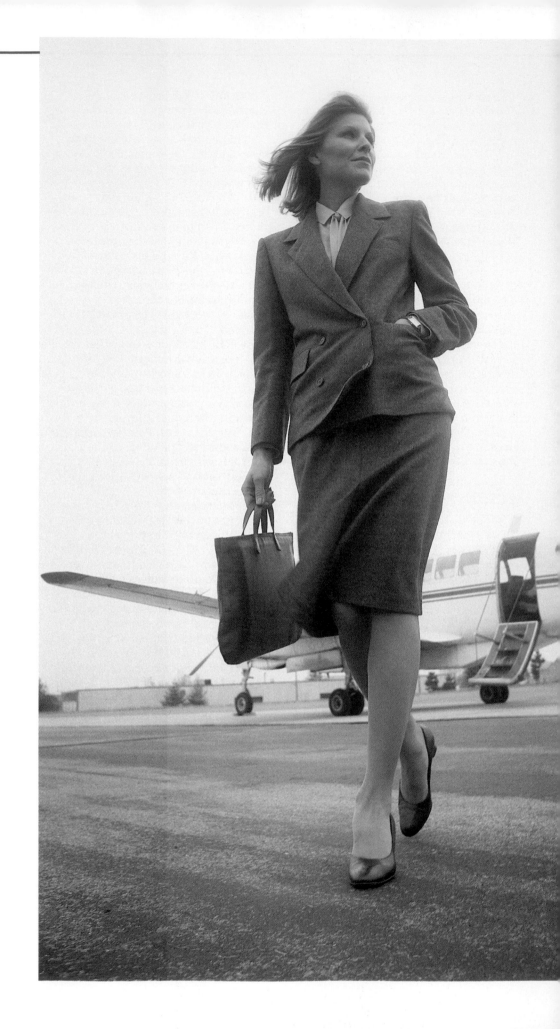

infection continues as long as it is worn, possibly up to a year or so after it is removed.

ENDING ENDOMETRIOSIS

For years, Elaine's menstrual periods caused her so little discomfort that she wondered what other women were talking about when they complained of terrible aches and pain. But one month, just prior to her period, 31-year-old Elaine woke up with unusually severe nagging pains in her abdomen. Her doctor prescribed medication and told her to return for a check-up in a few months.

Two days later, Elaine began hemorrhaging. She rushed to a local hospital, where a staff gynecologist examined her and diagnosed her problem as endometriosis, a disorder in which fragments of the uterine lining, which are usually shed through the vagina during menstruation, apparently become misdirected. These fragments are thought to back up into the fallopian tubes and spill out into the pelvic cavity, where they can become embedded on the outer wall of the uterus, the fallopian tubes or other pelvic organs.

The pain of endometriosis—

which can range from a constant ache during periods to a sudden jolt during intercourse—constitute only part of the trouble. Patches of tissue clogging the fallopian tubes can also result in infertility, although most women with this condition remain fertile.

An estimated eight million women in the United States have endometriosis. It afflicts only women between the ages of 25 and 45 who ovulate and menstruate regularly.

No one knows what causes this condition, but despite its seriousness, endometriosis can be overcome. Pregnancy is considered a solution, since the swollen endometrial tissue often shrinks and may even disappear in the absence of ovulation and menstruation. Menopause, too, often provides a spontaneous cure. A recently developed drug, Danazol, has been effective against endometriosis, but since it is a synthetic androgen, it can have masculinizing side effects, shrinking the breasts or deepening the voice. Those with endometriosis who bleed heavily should consider an iron supplement to guard against anemia. To relieve the pain, Yasuo Ishida, M.D., a St. Louis gynecologist, advises his patients to do exercises such as

---

The Bane of Career Women

Endometriosis, often dubbed "the career woman's disease," seems to affect a very narrow segment of the population— primarily women who have postponed or avoided pregnancy. Apparently, the longer a woman goes without interruption of her normal ovarian function—that is, without getting pregnant— the greater her chances of developing endometriosis. Some medical researchers have gone a step further, even suggesting that endometriosis is linked to personality traits commonly found in high-achieving career women. Veasy Buttram, M.D., of the Baylor College of Medicine, who conducted a study of 106 women, says the patients typically had "an intense desire to excel"

and were "tense perfectionists with demanding and specific goals." Most of them worked as secretaries or in professions like law or medicine.

Perhaps this ailment is yet another health problem doctors have dismissed as "psychological in nature."

Not *all* doctors, however. Joel T. Hargrove, M.D., a Tennessee researcher, has found that 78 percent of his endometriosis patients, who also have PMS, show an endocrine disorder. And John Rock, M.D., of the Harvard Medical School, dismisses the personality theory, saying, "I know of no data to confirm that endometriosis has anything at all to do with stress."

knee-chest bends, in which you kneel on hands and knees and lower your chest or head to the floor.

In some cases, surgery may be necessary to remove the swollen tissue. Yet Sherman Silber, M.D., a urologist and microsurgeon, says he believes surgery for correcting this condition is "overdone." According to Dr. Silber, studies have shown that for minimum to moderate adhesions with no blockage of the tubes, surgery is unnecessary. It's advisable to seek a second opinion if your doctor recommends surgery.

SEEKING HELP FOR FERTILITY PROBLEMS

On the surface, it seems easy enough. Millions of tiny tadpolelike sperm swim up a passageway, through an opening, then through a pear-shaped enclosure and into a tube. There, a wondrous happening occurs when one of these millions meets up with a small egg. United, the two become a tiny fertilized egg, which will then make its way slowly back down to the womb and grow into life.

But for all the supposed ease of this mating, there are countless obstacles that can throw the whole process awry. The fallopian tubes may be blocked due to scar tissue or infection. The sperm may be too weak to survive the 12-inch swim to meet the egg. Poor nutrition can cause a lack of sperm. Or some hostile mucus in the cervix, the opening to the uterus, may kill some sperm as they travel through it. Other problems abound.

The criterion of infertility is that a couple has been unable to conceive despite having unprotected intercourse for at least a year. Despite the modern tendency for couples to have small families or remain childless, plenty of couples want to conceive, but can't.

About 2.5 million couples visit doctors annually. An estimated 15 percent of all married couples are infertile.

For years, it was popularly considered to be the woman's "fault" if a couple was infertile. Actually, about 40 percent of infertility cases can be traced to the male.

Yet even recognizing when there is a problem and pinpointing the source of the difficulty can be tricky. Generally, experts say that 80 percent of women having regular intercourse will become pregnant within one year, and that increases to 90 percent by two years. So if you have not conceived by that time, there's a good chance something is out of whack.

Infertility counseling does not have a shot-in-the-dark feeling about

---

The Plummeting Sperm Count

Modern society and healthy sperm don't seem to mix. Sperm counts have vastly decreased over the past 30 years, contributing to the problem of infertility. Studies show that average sperm counts have gone from more than 145 million per milliliter in 1949 to just under 90 million in 1979. Toxic chemicals, such as polychlorinated biphenyls (PCBs), are believed to be one of the major culprits. Semen can become contaminated with chemicals via the food chain or through job exposure. Some animal studies have shown that vitamins A and C can help counter the effects of PCBs.

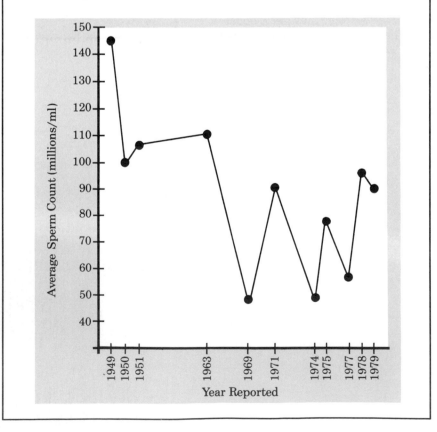

it but instead is a step-by-step process that begins with a medical history and a physical examination. From there, the focus first falls on the man, since it is usually easier to identify a male-related problem. A sample of semen is taken to determine if the volume and viability of the man's sperm are adequate to impregnate his partner.

Researchers have documented steadily declining sperm counts over the past three decades, primarily due to factors ranging from drugs to tight jeans or occupational exposure to lead (see "The Plummeting Sperm Count").

In women, the causes of infertility are a lot less clear-cut. Lack of ovulation can be the source. Blocked fallopian tubes may stop the egg from meeting the sperm. In addition, women who have been using birth control pills may find that their bodies do not automatically adjust when they stop taking the Pill because they want to have babies. Dr. Silber says that post-Pill infertility is more common than most people believe. "People feel assured of the reversability of the Pill, but there's no solid evidence that that's absolutely true," he says. "Think about it. In some women you have inhibition of ovulation for six, seven or more years. It seems likely that some women may not recover full ovulatory function."

In one study of 3,214 married women in New England, researchers found that 24.8 percent failed to conceive for 13 months or more after going off the Pill. Only 10.6 percent of women who had used other birth control methods failed to conceive in that period.

Whatever the problem, there are plenty of ways to reverse a couple's inability to conceive. One of the most "fertile" areas of recent study is the role of vitamins in aiding ovulation and bolstering sperm strength.

Masao Igarashi, M.D., a Japanese gynecologist, discovered that vitamin C worked in several cases where fertility drugs had not. The doctor gave vitamin C—by itself and in combination with the fertility drug clomiphene—to infertile women who habitually failed to ovulate and who had not responded to clomiphene therapy. In two out of five women, ovulation began with vitamin C alone. Vitamin C and clomiphene combined prompted ovulation in five out of five cases. In the case of one sterile woman who did not respond to drug treatment, Dr. Igarashi says a dosage of 400 milligrams of vitamin C daily "succeeded in induction of ovulation and conception. Afterwards, she delivered a normal baby at full term."

Two gynecologists found that high doses of vitamin B_6 were a successful treatment for infertile women who all shared one common problem—premenstrual tension. Joel Hargrove, M.D., of Columbia, Tennessee, and Guy E. Abraham, M.D., of Rolling Hills, California, conducted a study with 14 female patients who had been infertile from 18 months to seven years. After taking daily dosages of vitamin B_6 ranging from 100 to 800 milligrams, depending on how much was needed to relieve their PMS symptoms, 12 of 14 patients were finally able to conceive. Eleven became pregnant within the first six months of therapy. (This level of B_6 should be taken only under a doctor's supervision.)

Male fertility may get a boost from natural remedies, too. In Texas, Earl Dawson, Ph.D., measured the effects of a vitamin C preparation on 27 men between the ages of 25 and 38 who had been diagnosed as infertile. After 60 days, all 20 men who took the vitamin C preparation (which included calcium, magnesium and manganese) had impregnated their wives. None of the 7 men in the group not given vitamin C had.

To boost your fertility quotient, make sure you're getting proper nutrition and exercise. Controlling your weight and cutting back on smoking and alcohol helps, too. There are also lots of resources for help. The American Fertility Society has a number of pamphlets and a recommended reading list for couples; they may be obtained by writing the group at 1608 13th Avenue, South, Suite 101, Birmingham, AL 35256. Most of all, keep in mind that a couple needs to be supportive of each other to face and overcome this two-sided problem.

Tips to Aid Fertility

• Keep your weight close to normal. Extremes may affect the egg's monthly release from the ovary.

• Keep a record of menstrual cycles to help you figure out your fertile days.

• Have sexual intercourse every 24 to 48 hours during the fertile period. More frequent intercourse will decrease conception chances because sperm become depleted.

• Don't douche.

• Remain on your back with a pillow under the hips, with knees drawn up for 15 to 30 minutes after intercourse.

• Men can improve production of sperm by cutting back on alcohol, cigarettes and coffee, and maybe by wearing loose-fitting underwear.

• Try to relax! Physical and emotional stress can interfere with fertility, so keep the fun in your love life!

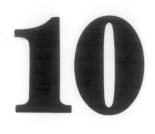

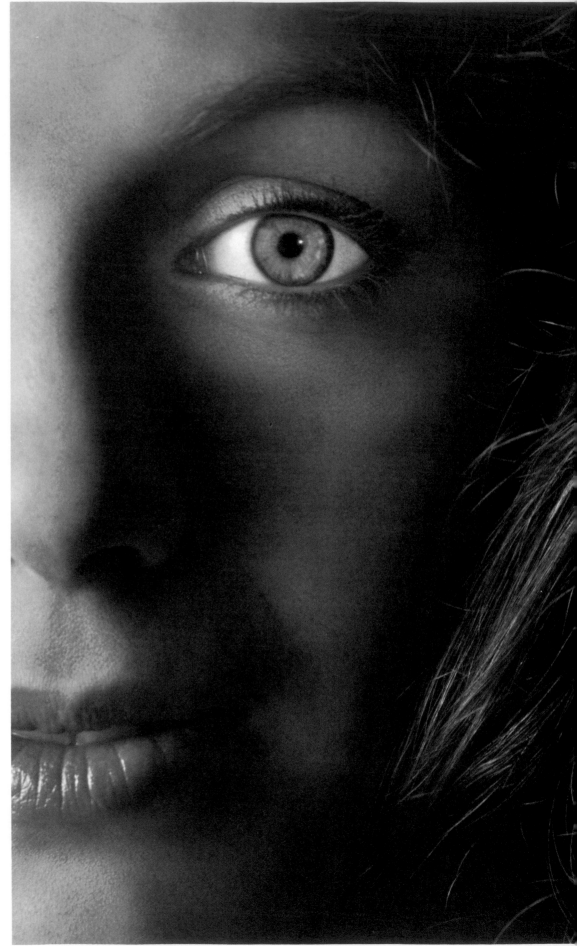

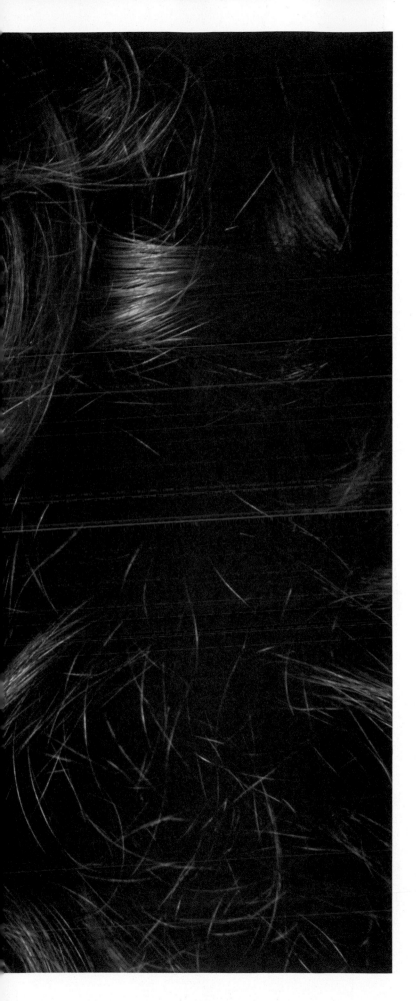

The Mind and the Senses

A sound body and a sound mind are one. If diet heals the body, then it also can heal the mind.

Stop for a moment, close your eyes and try to count the number of thoughts rushing through your brain. The first thought you count is the instruction you just received. Next, you might add the perception of your chair creaking. Then you'll be aware of your eyeballs moving underneath your eyelids, as though they are trying in the darkness to help you count. The memory of yesterday's lunch pops up. Soon, you realize that there is so much going on—a constant whir—that your brain's activities are impossible to keep track of. And these thoughts are only part of the commotion in your brain.

While you are thinking, your brain is working on the sly, performing behind the scenes to ensure that your body works smoothly, and that your perceptions are accurate. When you stub your toe, your brain lets you know it happened. If, when driving in the country, you catch the glorious sight of a group of deer bounding toward the woods, you owe the sight to your brain.

The brain functions well, with occasional lapses, in most people. But sometimes it misfires, causing a host of problems, including mental illness. In the past, these emotional and neurological problems were kept in the closet. But now, thankfully, problems with the brain more often are seen as correctable diseases than as tragic flaws. And nutrition is playing a vital role in treatment. Innovative psychotherapists are saying that nutritional health goes hand in hand with a healthy mind. Vitamins and minerals may play a bigger role in mental health than any Oedipal complex; they might have more effect on the senses than the aging process. Nutrition, in fact, may be the key to retaining a keen mind, along with good hearing and sharp eyesight.

DISSOLVING THOSE CLOUDS CALLED CATARACTS

Researchers have been testing the effectiveness of nutrition against eye diseases, and with good reason. Eye diseases are widespread among older people. In fact, 24.5 million Americans over age 60 suffer from cataracts alone.

Cataract is a generic term, derived from the Latin word for waterfall and used by doctors to describe any cloudy patch that mars the normally crystal-clear lens of the eye. Ideally, light should pass unobstructed through the lens and form a sharp image on the sensitive rear wall of the eye, known as the retina. But in an eye with a cataract, light strikes the cloudy patch and scatters aimlessly.

One cause of this problem, ironically, may be light itself. Just as direct sunlight can make your carpets fade while it brightens your rooms, light entering the eye not only delivers an image but also may cause undesirable chemical changes in the tissue. Certain by-products of those reactions, known as superoxides or free radicals, can attack a healthy lens and cause clouding.

Fortunately, vitamin C and vitamin E in the eye may act as "scavengers," intercepting the free radicals and neutralizing their effects.

That is the theory proposed by cataract specialists Shambhu Varma, Ph.D., and Richard D. Richards, Ph.D., of the University of Maryland Medical School in Baltimore. In an experiment, they took lenses from animals and bathed them in special solutions. Some of the solutions were then fortified with vitamin E, while others weren't. When the lenses were exposed to daylight, the vitamin-protected lenses suffered significantly less damage from superoxides than the unprotected lenses. In similar experiments, these two researchers found that vitamin C protects in the same way.

These Maryland physicians were not alone in their quest for a natural cataract treatment.

One prominent New Orleans ophthalmologist, Robert Azar, M.D., has made good nutrition a standard part of his care of cataract patients. He thinks that the right nutrients can halt or even reverse the problem.

People who approach Dr. Azar for removal of their clouded lenses are asked to start a supplement program of 1,000 to 1,500 milligrams of vitamin C a day, 15 to 30 milligrams of zinc and 200 to 400 I.U. of a water-soluble form of vitamin E. They're also urged to begin a diet low in fat and high in complex carbohydrates, a diet that stresses fish, fowl and fresh produce.

"Before we perform cataract surgery on anyone, we put them on our special diet program for two months," Dr. Azar says. "If their eyes begin to improve, we delay surgery

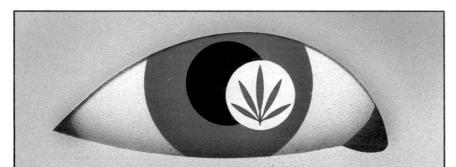

Marijuana for Glaucoma: Just Blowing Smoke

It began with reports in the late 1970s that smoking marijuana had helped a few persons with glaucoma feel better. Then others assumed pot might help them. Some people accused the government of withholding a valuable treatment by not making marijuana available and legal. Don't believe it. Anyone who tells you that the answer to glaucoma is spelled p-o-t is, well, just blowing smoke.

The flurry of attention and excitement over announcements that marijuana might be used to help relieve eye pressure has turned to disappointment. Keith Green, Ph.D., a professor of ophthalmology at the Medical College of Georgia in Augusta, says that marijuana "is totally unacceptable as a treatment for glaucoma because of the intolerable side effects." Besides, any relief that the drug provides is not found in all patients. Trying pot for glaucoma only gets you low.

for four more months. As long as their vision is improving, we keep putting off the operation. We've found that many people who stay on the diet don't have to go to surgery. Those who still need surgery tolerate the operation better."

In addition to zinc and vitamins C and E, the relationship between certain B vitamins and cataracts has intrigued several researchers. In a study of 173 patients at the Eye Foundation Hospital in Birmingham, Alabama, Harold W. Skalka, M.D., and Josef Prchal, M.D., noticed that riboflavin (vitamin B$_2$) and cloudless lenses seemed to go together. Twenty percent of their cataract patients under age 50 were deficient in riboflavin, as were 34 percent of their cataract patients over 50. But when they examined a group of 16 people over 50 who had good vision and clear lenses, every one of them had high levels of riboflavin in their blood.

"Riboflavin might not prevent cataracts," Dr. Skalka says, "but it may be able to help retard their formation."

GLAUCOMA DEMANDS EARLY TREATMENT

Like cataracts, glaucoma is a potentially blinding eye disease that attacks older people. The scary thing about glaucoma is that it sneaks up on you. Its often-overlooked symptoms are tunnel vision, poor vision in dim light, and rainbow-colored "halos" around lights. Drugs can control the disease, but there's no known cure.

An abnormally large buildup of pressure inside the eye (called intraocular pressure) is what causes glaucoma—and there's a possibility that vitamin C can lower that pressure and stem the disease. So far, researchers have found that healthy people who consume about 1,200 milligrams of vitamin C per day tend to have less pressure inside their eyes than people who consume only about 75 milligrams of the vitamin every day.

Thiamine (vitamin B$_1$) also may help glaucoma sufferers. A study by California ophthalmologist Edward R. Asregadoo, M.D., showed that people

Focus on Extended-Wear Lenses

Traditional contacts are great . . . except when you have to wander blindly from the bed to the bathroom each morning to put them in. But now there are extended-wear lenses that can stay in your eyes for up to 6 months. Great news! Are they safe?

Yes, says Robert Morrison, O.D., contact lens authority. Of more than 2,000 people he studied, 81 percent had no problem wearing the lenses anywhere from 2 weeks to 6 months without removing them. In addition, long-term lenses reduce the chances of developing an eye infection, because the lenses are handled less frequently. Unlike some other types of lenses, the extended-wear type can be used by people with astigmatism.

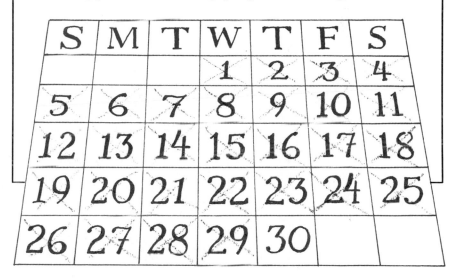

with glaucoma usually have lower amounts of thiamine in their blood.

It seems that while their diets contained roughly the same amount of thiamine as the diets of people with good vision, their bodies apparently couldn't make use of it. Dr. Asregadoo thinks that people who are genetically prone to glaucoma can benefit from taking large doses of thiamine. (But don't take more than 50 milligrams a day without your doctor's okay.)

In his practice in Walnut Creek, California, Dr. Asregadoo has had excellent results with vitamins. "My patients say they feel generally better with moderately high doses of vitamins B and C, and none of them in the last 12 years needed surgery for control of the intraocular pressure."

A LIFETIME OF GOOD HEARING

Add hearing loss to the litany of ills brought on by cigarette smoking. Studies conducted at the University of Washington, Seattle, and Cairo University in Egypt show a correlation between puffing cigarettes and not being able to hear. The results are shown in the chart: Smokers show considerably more deafness than nonsmokers. It is believed that cigarette smoke works to clog up the ears and increase pressure, resulting in hearing loss.

Helen Keller, who was both blind and deaf, said in later life that deafness was a worse affliction than blindness. The loss of hearing cuts a person off from the world around him—the whispered secrets and laughs of joy as well as the ringing phone and pounding hammer.

Why should someone be deprived of this precious sense? Some researchers are rapidly putting together the pieces of a theory pointing to general stress as an important cause of hearing problems.

Gordon R. Bienvenue, Ph.D., an audiologist at the State University of New York, New Paltz, believes that noise itself does not directly cause hearing loss, but that noise is a form of stress which, along with other types of stress, can contribute to the problem.

Martin Robinette, Ph.D., a professor of audiology at the University of Utah, has found that the combined stresses of alcohol in your system and loud sounds is particularly bad. People listening to loud music while drinking suffer temporary hearing loss that has been measured. Dr. Robinette got volunteers to take the equivalent of four drinks over a two-hour period and to listen to loud music. He found their hearing levels to be below those of volunteers who weren't intoxicated, but who heard the same music. Such an exposure may eventually lead to a more permanent hearing loss.

NUTRITION ENHANCES SOUND

If it's surprising that stress can deaden your ability to hear, it's even more surprising that positive nutrition and general health improvement can preserve hearing. There is the beginning of hard evidence that a good diet works. James T. Spencer, Jr., M.D., an ear specialist in Charleston, West Virginia, found that he was able to improve his own hearing after he stopped eating wheat and white sugar entirely, and also drastically reduced his intake of fats. He lost 14 pounds, saw his cholesterol and triglyceride levels go down, and was surprised to find that most of his ability to hear was restored.

Dr. Spencer, who is an associate clinical professor of otolaryngology at West Virginia University School of Medicine, has examined hundreds of patients for nutritional as well as hearing problems. In the *West Virginia Medical Journal* he reported that 87 percent of his patients with hearing problems were prediabetic and 80 percent were obese. He advised them to practice "good basic nutrition," and those who followed his advice enjoyed what he called a "phenomenal gain in hearing."

Another audiologist also investigating the connection between nutri-

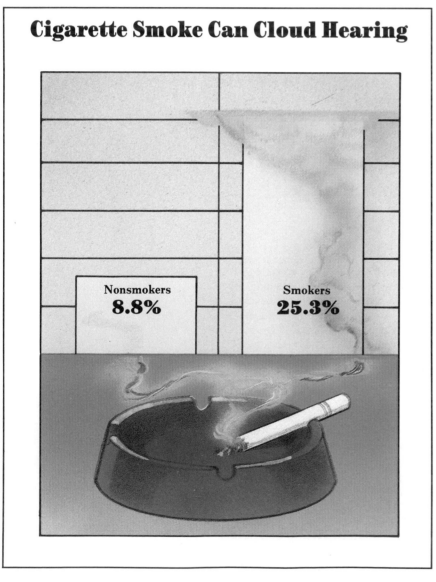

Cigarette Smoke Can Cloud Hearing

Nonsmokers
8.8%

Smokers
25.3%

tion and hearing is Paul Yanick, Ph.D. Along with several physicians, he runs a clinic in New York City. There they treat hearing problems holistically. One of the doctrines they hold true is the relationship between diet and hearing. In fact, they believe that many of the 36 million Americans who suffer from hearing loss can be helped only if they realize that this loss is often caused by poor diet. What they suggest—particularly for people who have very high levels of cholesterol and triglycerides in their blood—is switching to a diet high in raw vegetables and fruits. Lecithin, known to reduce levels of blood fats, also may be recommended. Finally, the New York clinic strongly endorses the value of exercise. People taking these suggestions often get a dramatic improvement in their hearing. Those with tinnitus (ear noises) often report complete relief.

HEARING LOSS REVERSED

Why does improving diet and nutrition work to reverse hearing loss?

"Basically, the ear can have three main problems," Dr. Yanick explains. "One, not receiving enough oxygen. Two, not receiving the proper balance of nutrients because of circulatory problems and/or inherent biochemical and nutritional imbalances. Three, not receiving enough glucose, or blood sugar.

"The ear has been found to have the highest energy requirements of the whole body, and its principal energy source is glucose. Without glucose, the cells can't function and the hearing process can't occur. If it does occur, it will be on a very minimal basis—you'll hear, but you won't hear things clearly," he continues.

"White sugar, white bread, fats, caffeine, salt, smoking and lack of exercise—they all work to unbalance glucose levels, clog circulation and cut off oxygen to the ear as well as the whole body. Good diet, exercise and the proper individualized nutritional supplements can usually correct any of these problems.

"The nutritional supplements a person requires depend on that individual's nutritional needs and on how

various systems of the body are interrelating with the hearing mechanism," Dr. Yanick says.

"The B vitamins are important to nerve function, and the ear is composed of a sense organ and a nerve. The B vitamins are known to help people under stress. They also play a major role in glucose metabolism, which is important to the ear.

"B_6 is known to act as a natural diuretic to stabilize the balance of electrolytes that are found in the inner ear fluids. In certain cases of electrolyte imbalance, a person might want to take B_6 three times a day.

"Vitamin A is also very important. The cilia cells in the ear, which are the cells that give rise to hearing, are dependent upon vitamin A. Vitamin A should be taken with lecithin, because it's fat soluble and lecithin helps the system digest and assimilate it.

"Vitamins C and E and the trace mineral selenium are also important because they're antioxidants," says Dr. Yanick. "They increase the amount of oxygen that gets to the cells. Any vitamin that increases oxygen is important."

GOOD FOOD, GOOD HEARING

And when it comes to taking nutritional supplements, Dr. Yanick practices what he preaches. He reversed his own hearing loss and eliminated severe tinnitus with diet and exercise. "I take a select mixture of multivitamins in the morning," he says, "and if I'm under a lot of stress, I'll take vitamin C in the afternoon. I also take minerals such as chromium and potassium."

But his main source of vitamins and minerals isn't food supplements—it's food. Natural food. He completely changed his diet, and the benefits were immediate.

"Within a month and a half my hearing stabilized and hasn't gotten worse since. Since that time, I've been on a high-natural-carbohydrate, low-fat, medium-protein diet. I've eliminated all processed, refined grains and sugar. I eat a lot of raw vegetables and fruits."

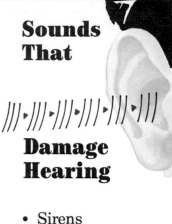

Sounds That

$$\rangle\rangle\rangle \blacktriangleright \rangle\rangle\rangle \blacktriangleright \rangle\rangle\rangle \blacktriangleright \rangle\rangle\rangle \blacktriangleright \rangle\rangle\rangle$$

Damage Hearing

- Sirens
- Discos
- Motorcycles
- Power mowers
- Rock concerts
- Traffic
- Snowmobiles
- Chain saws
- Airplanes
- Gunfire
- Drills

A Map of Your Taste Buds

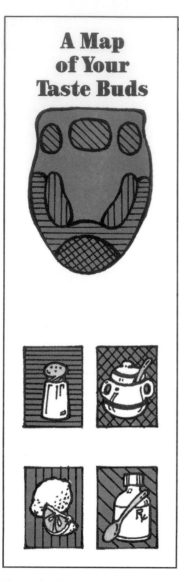

Taste buds aren't spread randomly around the tongue, but are grouped according to specific tastes. Though some people would swear the buds that sense sweets cover their whole tongue, the sweet-sensing buds are only at the tip. The salt sensors cover a horseshoe-shaped swath near the front of the tongue, bordered by the buds that tell you a lemon is sour. Finally, alone in the back where they belong are the buds that register bitterness.

A PROBLEM OF TASTE

"There are probably ten million people in the United States who have taste problems," says Robert Henkin, M.D., who runs the Center for Molecular Nutrition and Sensory Disorders at Georgetown University Medical Center in Washington, D.C. Hypogeusia, the scientific name for taste loss, is not itself a disease, says Dr. Henkin. For example, we all know taste loss can accompany a bad cold. And nutritional factors also may be involved. Zinc deficiency is one cause. But, Dr. Henkin notes, "Copper deficiency can influence it, vitamin A deficiency can influence it, as well as deficiencies in vitamins B_{12} and B_6."

In one study, Allan Shatzman, Ph.D., a biochemist associated with the taste center, and Dr. Henkin set out to define more clearly the effects of zinc therapy on the sense of taste.

"We reported only one case, but he is representative of a number of taste loss cases we've handled," says Dr. Henkin.

Each day of the study, samples of the patient's saliva were collected from the parotid gland, which secretes the majority of the protein found in saliva. The samples were analyzed for their content of zinc and gustin. "Gustin is the salivary protein which contains significant amounts of zinc," Dr. Henkin explains. "Seventy-five to 80 percent of the zinc in saliva is bound to this protein."

The patient's saliva was compared with saliva from normal, healthy people. Both the healthy saliva and the saliva taken from the patient with taste loss were first broken down into separate components, or fractions, as the scientists call them, of the whole saliva from the parotid gland. "In normal people, and with patients with hypogeusia, all these fractions are about the same, except for fraction II," Dr. Henkin says. "Fraction II is that part of the saliva which contains gustin, the zinc-containing protein. We could clearly see that something was different in fraction II of the patient's saliva."

While the zinc content of all the saliva of patients with taste loss may be about half the normal amount, the deficiency is particularly apparent with respect to fraction II of the saliva. There the levels of gustin (and therefore zinc) are as low as *one-fifth* of normal. Gustin and the zinc it contains appear to be crucial factors in normal taste.

That suspicion was confirmed when the test patient was given zinc supplements. As treatment with zinc proceeded, the levels of zinc and gustin in the patient's saliva increased, and his ability to taste improved dramatically.

"The patient reached a maximum ability to taste on day 12," Dr. Henkin says. "The return to normal taste followed by three days the return to normal biochemistry in the saliva."

MORE THAN TASTE BUDS

Dr. Henkin believes that while this evidence indicates that zinc works to maintain the sense of taste by maintaining normal taste bud function in the mouth, zinc may also affect taste centers in the brain, where information from taste buds is received and processed. However, he says, "The majority of patients we see who have taste problems have biochemical problems that are influenced by changes in saliva or the taste buds directly, not in the brain."

Though treatment with zinc helps correct the taste problems of many of Dr. Henkin's patients, he believes that the original cause of their problems is not an inadequate diet, but the way their bodies utilize the zinc in the food they eat. "These people may be taking in the same amount of zinc as you or I, but they don't absorb it or utilize it properly," he says. Abnormalities in the way their bodies utilize zinc may require that they take in more zinc than others in the hope that this increase can overcome these abnormalities.

Even considered in terms of the government's Recommended Dietary Allowances, which set the adult zinc requirement at 15 milligrams a day, great portions of the American population are not getting enough zinc to meet their needs. The typical American is believed to consume

Sunburgers—A Taste of Zinc

Makes 4 servings

½ teaspoon olive oil
1 cup sunflower seeds
1½ cup chick-peas, cooked until very soft and drained
1 teaspoon olive oil
1 egg

1 tablespoon stock or water
1 teaspoon ground ginger
1 teaspoon coriander
2 tablespoons parsley (optional)

Place the olive oil and sunflower seeds in a heavy skillet over medium-high heat. Stir constantly until the seeds brown. Transfer to a food processor or blender. Add all other ingredients and process into a paste.

Form the mixture into 4 patties. Bake for 10 minutes on a lightly oiled pan. Turn burgers over and bake 5 minutes longer.

Serve on whole wheat rolls.

between 10 and 15 milligrams of zinc a day. Among older people, zinc intake is often less than half of the RDA. Older people, not surprisingly, also commonly suffer taste loss.

What this wholesale deadening of the nation's taste buds does to our cuisine is anyone's guess. Are some people's palates so dull that they *can't* distinguish anything more subtle than pretzels and cotton candy? Is that why blatant seasonings like salt and sugar dominate our preparation of food? Could be.

FOODS TASTE SWEETER

A study of young women reviewed their zinc status by analyzing their blood, saliva, hair and diet. Their zinc status was judged to be normal, and they were given different concentrations of zinc supplements. There was no change in the women's ability to detect three of the four basic tastes, sourness, bitterness and saltiness. But for women receiving 50 milligrams of zinc a day, there was a significant increase in their ability to taste sweetness.

Another study recorded an improvement in older people's ability to taste sweetness with zinc supplementation, plus an improve-

ment in the ability to taste salt. But the improvements were not statistically significant—perhaps, the authors of the study speculated, because the people were receiving only 15 milligrams of zinc supplements a day.

In any case, the interesting thing about those two studies is the improvement in the ability to taste sweetness recorded in both. The more sensitive you are to sweetness, the less sugar you need to achieve the same taste. Getting adequate zinc might be one way to cut back our intake of sugar.

Consider eating foods such as fish, lima beans, liver, nuts and sunflower and pumpkin seeds—all good sources of zinc. Also consider taking zinc supplements if necessary. Eating, after all, was meant to be one of life's true pleasures. So enjoy.

SELF-STARVATION AND BINGING OVERCOME

We live in the land of plenty, but some among us are starving. These are not poor children in rags wandering through inner-city ghettos or across hills thick with black dust from strip-mined coal. These are people, mostly women, from all-American families. They live in spacious ranch homes in the suburbs or comfortable townhouses in the nice sections of cities. They don't waste away from lack of food. They suffer in the face of abundance.

They are the victims of bulimia and anorexia nervosa. Theirs is a problem of unrealistic self-images. They look in the mirror and see themselves as fat and imperfect, no matter how thin they are.

Even though they crave food, anorexics starve themselves until they begin to look like skeletons. Bulimics are not necessarily emaciated, but they fight calories as fiercely as anorexics. They binge on huge amounts of food and then purge the calories from their bodies by vomiting or taking large quantities of laxatives. Some physicians and psychiatrists are now combining the diseases under one label, bulimarexia, because they seem to go hand in hand. In fact, says William Philpott, M.D., a psychiatrist who is director of the Philpott Medical Center in St. Petersburg, Florida, "I have never seen a bulimic who at one time or another hadn't been anorexic."

The diseases have definite psychological factors, but now, very effective treatments use proper nutrition and psychotherapy to cure bulimarexia.

FOODS TRIGGER THE NEED

Unlike most doctors, Dr. Philpott believes that bulimarexia is not a purely psychological problem. Instead it may be a biological reaction to foods. He says that certain foods—which vary from person to person—cause an enzymatic reaction in the body that triggers the desire to go hungry. This self-starvation in turn sets off the production of endorphins (natural, addictive "narcotics") in the body. The anorexic becomes addicted to the good feelings endorphins produce, and continues in a pattern of self-starvation. As a result, brain chemistry is thrown out of balance, thus distorting the sense of self-perception, says Dr. Philpott. This false sense of self may explain why anorexics, who are little more than skin and bones, can look in a mirror and see themselves as fat.

This food-reaction theory is supported by Hans Heubner, M.D., who wrote in the newsletter of the American Anorexia/Bulimia Association, Inc. that the "relentless weight loss, and fear of getting fat, can be understood in terms of an addiction to the body's natural painkiller, the endorphins, and a need of the mind to maintain this addiction."

Dr. Philpott's first treatment goal is to find the foods that are causing the problem. He has his patients spend the first week of treatment eating only foods that they previously rarely ate. These usually don't produce a reaction. The patients then return to single-food meals of more common foods—the

The Story of an Anorexic

She's 19 years old now, and trying to get back on her feet after spending almost a quarter of her life on the anorexia merry-go-round. Her first period of great weight loss started when she was 15. She decided that 90 pounds was her maximum weight and then dropped to 89 pounds, just to be certain she wouldn't go over. Eighty-nine became the new goal, so she dropped another pound. Then another. The cycle continued ever downward, fueled by self-starvation and obsessive running—if she ate 2 carrots she forced herself to run 2 miles. When she dropped to 80 pounds she began to have dizzy spells. She was sent to a children's hospital for 2 weeks. For the next 2 years she was "fine"—no serious anorexic behavior. Then, after a period of emotional stress, the anorexic behavior returned. She felt powerful when she starved herself. It was her way of having perfect control of herself. She cut starches and fats from her diet. Then she ate nothing but vegetables. Sometimes she would go 3 days without eating. Coffee fueled her and killed the hunger pangs. Finally she ended up in the Stanford Medical Center for 6 weeks. She is an outpatient now—4 years after first entering a hospital for anorexia—better, but not cured.

ones they liked before they got sick. Dr. Philpott watches their reactions to these single-food meals. If they exhibit signs of anorexia, he knows the food is one that produces adverse reactions. It is then added to the list of foods requiring caution. Dr. Philpott says that once they are well, most anorexics can return to eating the foods which previously triggered anorexic behavior. But to avoid further reactions, they must not eat any one food more than once every four days.

Once the problem foods have been identified, Dr. Philpott works to bring the woman's vitamin and mineral status back to a healthy level—an essential first step before psychological therapy can do any good. Otherwise, the patient's psychological condition will deteriorate along with her physical condition. A study conducted by doctors at the University of Cincinnati College of Medicine showed just how interrelated the mind and body are.

Four adolescent girls who had lost a mean 41 percent of their body weight (equal to dropping from 120 pounds to 71 pounds) were hospitalized with anorexia. Because of their resistance to all treatments, nutritionally balanced intravenous solutions were used to restore the girls' nutrition over an average period of 25 days. The vitamins did their job and the patients' mental health improved along with their bodies, as the nutrients flowed through their system. With psychotherapy and good nutrition, all of the girls remained well after follow-ups of 5 to 16 months.

If the patient is bulimic, Dr. Philpott uses behavior modification to get her out of the habit of vomiting. The therapy goes like this: The offending food is named, the patient gets an urge to vomit, and a mild electric shock (not enough to cause a seizure) is administered. The shock gives the patient a negative association with vomiting. This treatment is repeated four times a minute, 15 minutes a day, for 10 to 15 days. By this time, says Dr. Philpott, the patient is usually well on the way to recovery. The patient continues to practice behavior modification at home by thinking about a particular

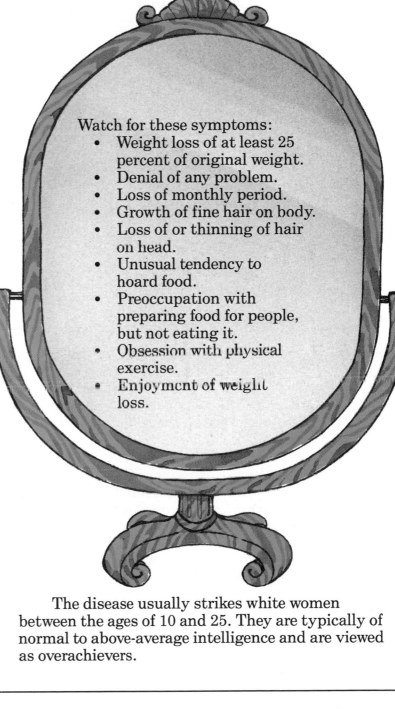

How Thin Is Too Thin?
Warning Signs of Anorexia Nervosa

Watch for these symptoms:
- Weight loss of at least 25 percent of original weight.
- Denial of any problem.
- Loss of monthly period.
- Growth of fine hair on body.
- Loss of or thinning of hair on head.
- Unusual tendency to hoard food.
- Preoccupation with preparing food for people, but not eating it.
- Obsession with physical exercise.
- Enjoyment of weight loss.

The disease usually strikes white women between the ages of 10 and 25. They are typically of normal to above-average intelligence and are viewed as overachievers.

food and holding her breath until any negative feelings disappear. In time, if the treatment works, the desire to vomit will cease.

However, bulimarexia is not subject to a quick fix. Retuning the body is only the first step in treatment. Long-term support is usually necessary. The psychological aspects of the disease are very important and, like the physical symptoms, should be treated by a doctor.

Steven Levenkron, a New York City psychotherapist, says of bulimarexics: "They want someone to take care of them, someone who's assertive, who knows what they are doing and who's sensitive and understanding to what they're going through." The parents usually are unable to cope with such bizarre behavior from their child. That's where the therapist comes in. "The girls need direction. And they will accept your advice if you've succeeded in gaining their trust," says Levenkron.

OVERCOMING SENILITY

The young look to their parents and grandparents for sage advice, because years of ups and downs have given them a good understanding of the world. Their advice is sound until senility strikes. Then everyone is deprived of this precious resource.

Senility can reverse personalities. A once kind woman can turn into a demanding, irascible crank. A man who had a sharp memory when young may be reduced to not even remembering the phone number he's had for 30 years. Senile people often lose their ability to take care of themselves and can become completely dependent on others. An estimated 10 percent of Americans over 65 suffer from some form of intellectual impairment. We generally accept this mental deterioration as an unfortunate part of aging, like hearing loss and gray hair. Sometimes families, though devoted, are unable to meet the senile parent's special needs. Reluctantly, they book them into a retirement or nursing home.

This rather drastic step is unfortunate, because in many cases, the senility isn't permanent at all. Perhaps as many as 20 percent of the roughly three million Americans diagnosed as senile suffer from intellectual afflictions that are actually *reversible*. Among other causes, drugs and poor nutrition can bring about the problem, rather than mental deterioration.

Prescription drugs are perhaps the most devastating culprits. The typical senior citizen takes between four and seven drugs each day. Though the elderly comprise only 11 percent of the population, they suffer more than 50 percent of all drug side

---

Dr. Diamond's Fascinating Rats

Many people believe that as we grow old our minds automatically shift into neutral. It would seem that we lose the capacity for growth, that our natural curiosity is gone, that our inner vision has become myopic.

Bored, the mind just shuts off. Is this mental deterioration an inevitable part of aging? No, says Marian Diamond, Ph.D., a California neuroanatomist, who challenges some of the myths regarding the aging brain. After experimenting with laboratory rats, she has determined that the brain's decline may simply result from a bland and boring life.

She began her study by placing some young rats in an enriched environment and others in a nonstimulating environment. She gave the first group lots of toys, which were varied every day. When examined, the brains of these stimulated animals were larger and more chemically active than the brains of the normal lab animals, living in a small, boring cage.

Now you can't always apply animal studies to people. But in this case, common sense dictates that you probably can. Boredom and a lack of stimulation make a person of any age boring and unstimulating. An unchallenged, unoccupied mind often turns inward, dwelling on the past, on losses or on current aches and pains. The result is often apathy and, more serious, depression. Staying outgoing and active is the best way to remain young at heart and in mind.

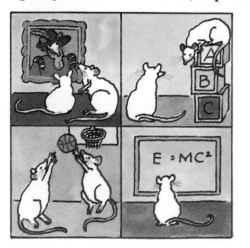
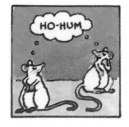

effects. This is due, in part, to aging kidneys which are unable to process medication as easily as they used to. The result is that the drugs build up in the body and cause side effects that in the elderly are commonly associated with senility—anxiety, slurred speech and irritability.

Sedatives, tranquilizers and sleeping pills—as well as any other psychoactive drug—probably cause most of these problems. "They interfere with neurotransmitters, the chemicals that regulate brain function," says Richard W. Besdine, M.D., a specialist in geriatrics. "And they weaken coordination between the parts of the brain. These drugs have the potential to cause intellectual impairment in a person of any age, and the elderly are the most vulnerable. Old brains are more sensitive to the confusion-inducing side effects of psychoactive drugs," continues Dr. Besdine.

If someone you know is showing signs of senility—disorientation, memory loss, depression, irritability—be certain that the problem isn't simply drug related before institutionalizing the person. It could be that the "symptoms of senility" are side effects, and more serious than the problems the drugs are supposed to cure. A doctor probably can suggest an alternative. Once the harmful drugs are eliminated from the body, it might be desirable to start adding some vitamins.

VITAMINS: THE SIMPLE CURE

Of course, elderly people need to maintain good levels of all the essential vitamins and minerals, but research shows that the B vitamins may play an especially essential role in maintaining a sound mind.

Niacin has been shown to have a direct effect on "senility." Niacin deficiency can result in depression, irritability, memory loss, insomnia, mental confusion, and distractibility—all considered symptoms of senility. Researchers at the University of Saskatchewan in Canada gave ten senile people niacin—with good results. Five of the ten recovered completely from "senility" after the niacin therapy and two others had "marked

Causes of Mock Senility

Many times a patient will be diagnosed as irreversibly senile when the problem is actually reversible. Below are some of the causes of false senility.

Drugs
Lithium
Barbiturates
Atropine
Bromides

Heavy Metals
Mercury
Arsenic
Lead
Thalium

Toxins
Air pollution
Alcohol

Diseases
Epilepsy
Multiple sclerosis
Wilson's disease
Anemia
Pellagra
Hypoglycemia
Meningitis
SLE
Trauma
Encephalitis

improvement." The B vitamins thiamine and B_{12} also play a crucial role. The deficiency symptoms of both vitamins include—you guessed it—the frequent signs of senility: fatigue, insomnia, irritability, depression and confusion.

The elderly become deficient in these and other vitamins for a variety of reasons, perhaps the primary one being a change in diet. Some older people just simply lose interest in eating because they are lonely, poor or unable to get to a grocery store, or because they lose their teeth, as well as their senses of taste and smell. It takes effort to overcome these setbacks. Zinc has been shown to stimulate the appetite. And common sense tells us that companionship at dinner will make the meal seem a lot more attractive than a lonely session in front of a television. Nutritious meals can be simple *and* easy to prepare. Try cottage cheese topped with fresh fruit and wheat germ, or tuna surrounded by lettuce and fresh vegetables, to get the nutrition you need. A chicken breast and a potato will bake in the oven just about as quickly and easily as a TV dinner. Coffee and tea deplete the body of thiamine, so substitute fresh juice or herb tea whenever possible.

While good eating habits will surely make you feel better, it also might be wise to take a B complex supplement if you think you are vitamin deficient. At least take the government's Recommended Dietary Allowance, as listed on the label. You might have to take two a day to keep up.

NONDRUG CONTROLS FOR EPILEPSY

"There's going to be a revolution in the methods of treating epilepsy over the next 20 years." That's what J. O. McNamara, M.D., believes. He's the director of the epilepsy center at the Veterans' Administration Medical Center in Durham, North Carolina, and he has been working on this problem for years.

Epilepsy can result from a brain injury before or at the time of birth, very high fevers during early childhood and infectious diseases such as mumps or measles. Vitamin and mineral deficiencies, low blood sugar, chemical imbalances in the body or even brain tumors could be at the root of the disorder.

Regardless of the cause, treatment often involves the continual use

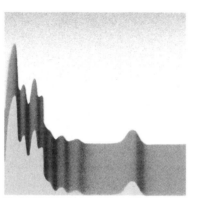

Normal person

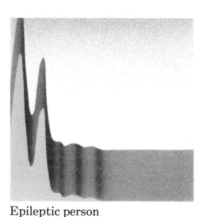

Epileptic person

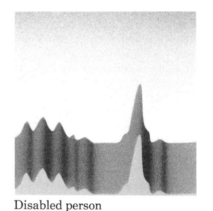

Disabled person

BRAIN WAVES DURING SLEEP

Relaxing the Seizures of Epilepsy

M. B. Sterman, Ph.D., chief of neuro-psychology research at the Veterans' Administration Medical Center in Sepulveda, California, uses biofeedback to treat patients with drug-resistant epilepsy.

"The procedure eventually leads," says Dr. Sterman, "to suppression of abnormal brain activity." A feedback display (examples of brain wave patterns are illustrated above) indicates a proper response. In this way a specific anticonvulsant "brain state" can be achieved.

"The results in my laboratory and elsewhere show that biofeedback is effective in 70 percent of the people studied," says Dr. Sterman.

Francis Forster, M.D., now retired, was a neurologist at the Veterans' Administration Hospital in Madison, Wisconsin. He also used a behavioral approach to help patients with reflex epilepsy, where seizures are brought on by everyday activities.

"We conditioned the patient so that the thing which triggered his attacks became innocuous," said Dr. Forster. "For example, if a certain piece of music caused a seizure, we reproduced it in the lab. Then we played that same melody over and over as the patient returned to consciousness. We continued to play it until it no longer evoked the negative response," he explained.

of anticonvulsive drugs, which eliminate or reduce the number of seizures in the majority of patients. However, many must learn to live with unpleasant side effects. Some 20 percent—400,000 people—find that drugs don't help at all.

In the revolution predicted by Dr. McNamara, natural treatments will earn a place alongside drug treatments—to the benefit of all.

"The importance of diet in regulating seizures is starting to come out," says Dr. McNamara. "And I think we are going to find out that nutrition plays a more important role in seizure control than anyone might have previously suspected. I'm very happy about the results we're getting."

For Dr. McNamara, those results involve the use of choline in the treatment of a type of epilepsy called complex partial seizures (CPS). The doctor selected four patients with CPS whose drug therapy was not working. During the four-month study, each patient was given choline along with his existing drug regimen. Doses started at 4 grams per day and were gradually increased to 12 or 16 grams per day by the third month (an extreme amount, to be taken only under the direction of a physician).

"Our principal finding," says Dr. McNamara, "was that a marked increase in plasma [blood] choline concentrations was associated with shorter seizures and less postseizure fatigue." The patients, too, considered themselves much improved and expressed resentment when the choline was discontinued after the study.

CERTAIN NUTRIENTS QUELL SEIZURES

In addition to choline, epilepsy researchers have found manganese also to be vital to seizure control. Yukio Tanaka, Ph.D., in work at the trace element laboratory at St. Mary's Hospital in Montreal, first suspected this connection. Based on this suspicion, he found that a little boy suffering from convulsive disorders that did not respond to medication had half the normal amount of manganese that he should have.

Enough of the mineral was given

Food Sources of Manganese

Food	Portion	Manganese (mcg.)
Wheatena	1 cup	1,997
Oatmeal	1 cup	1,369
Wheat germ	1 tbsp.	1,235
Shredded wheat cereal	1 cup	1,075
Spinach	½ cup	884
Collard greens	½ cup	601
Turnip greens	½ cup	395
Kale	½ cup	377
Broccoli	½ cup	346
Mustard greens	½ cup	342
Beans, lima	½ cup	276
Beans, snap, green	½ cup	275
Chicken liver	3 oz.	255
Peas, sweet	½ cup	226
Puffed rice cereal	1 cup	210
Banana	1 medium	173
Prunes	5 medium	93
Corn	½ cup	80

NOTE: Vegetables are uncooked.

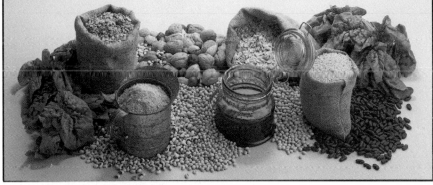

to the boy to raise his blood levels to normal. When that happened, his condition was noticeably improved. He had fewer seizures, and his gait, speech and learning were all better than before treatment started.

AN ANTIDOTE TO INJURY

L. James Willmore, M.D., a neuroscientist with the University of Texas Medical School in Houston, may have found a possible solution to the problem of epilepsy resulting from a head injury.

He explains that a blow to the head causes internal bleeding, and the ruptured red blood cells leak iron. This, in turn, leads to the formation of hydrogen peroxide, which is damaging to brain tissue. Dr. Willmore theorized that selenium and vitamin E, which are both antioxidant nutrients, may help prevent posttraumatic epilepsy.

Using rats, Dr. Willmore duplicated the condition that may occur in people after a head injury. Injections of selenium and vitamin E prevented epilepsy from occurring in 72 percent of the rats. In another group of rats given no treatment, only 6 percent escaped epilepsy.

NEW THERAPIES FOR SCHIZOPHRENIA

Schizophrenia is a broad mental illness. The afflicted lose touch with reality. They hear voices that don't exist and see things that aren't really there. The schizophrenic's thoughts make sense to the schizophrenic, but not to anyone else.

It seems to flitter through populations randomly. Yet, a young man growing up in western Ireland stands a 1 in 25 chance of being hospitalized with schizophrenia sometime in his life, while an American's chances are only 1 in 100. Like Ireland, northern Sweden and countries in eastern Europe also seem to have a high incidence of schizophrenia. The disease can come and go, and is believed to fade with old age. Oddly,

Schizophrenia Causes Now Identified and Treated

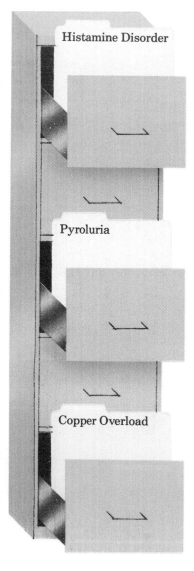

Histamine Disorder

Pyroluria

Copper Overload

One doctor who believes that schizophrenia is caused by a biochemical imbalance in the body is Carl Pfeiffer, M.D., Ph.D., the director of the Brain Bio Center in Skillman, New Jersey.

Dr. Pfeiffer calls schizophrenia a "biochemical wastebasket." Into that wastebasket, he says, have been thrown a variety of diseases, all of which were once thought to be schizophrenia. Dr. Pfeiffer has turned that wastebasket into a filing cabinet. He believes that he has isolated the remaining biochemical abnormalities that cause schizophrenia. And *nutrition can treat them all.*

One of them is pyroluria. In this disease, a person eliminates abnormally large amounts of the chemical kryptopyrrole. Unfortunately, on its way out, kryptopyrrole grabs onto zinc and B_6, both of which are crucial to normal brain function. The result is very low body levels of those nutrients—and schizophrenia. The treatment, however, is simple: replace B_6 and zinc. And the cure is almost automatic—95 percent recover.

Sixty percent of schizophrenics suffer from a histamine disorder, according to Dr. Pfeiffer. One of the functions of histamine is as a neurotransmitter, a chemical that relays information in the brain. But when histamine levels rise to high or dip too low, the brain can relay wrong information.

For schizophrenics with high histamine, Dr. Pfeiffer prescribes calcium, zinc and manganese. The treatment also includes the amino acid methionine.

"For patients with low histamine, large doses of niacin and vitamin C are usually effective," he explains. He also gives them zinc to lower their copper levels. "Copper and zinc are biological antagonists. When one comes in, the other goes out," says Dr. Pfeiffer.

if it develops later in life, it seems to strike those who were born during the late winter and early spring more than people who were born at other times of the year.

The intensity of the disease may vary from one person to another. But treatment, until recently, did not. Even today, it's standard to treat schizophrenics with psychoanalysis or with antipsychotic drugs, if they are treated at all. The results have been marginal at best. But now convincing evidence exists which shows that schizophrenia may be less an unexplainable mental curse than a simple reaction to certain foods.

A PROMISING TREATMENT

Prostaglandins, which are made from essential fatty acids, are present in every cell in the body. They appear to be the key regulators of every cell and organ. So it's not surprising that they may help some schizophrenics.

There are three main groupings of prostaglandins, but one, PG1, seems to be particularly related to schizophrenia. A good source of PG1 is evening primrose oil. A researcher in York, England, treated schizophrenics for 16 weeks with a combination of evening primrose oil and penicillin (which does not interfere with the synthesis of PG1). Of six "severe chronic schizophrenics," none became worse during treatment, and two showed striking improvement.

One patient, a woman, had been aggressive and uncooperative in the hospital, calling the police about once a week to accuse the staff of various crimes and writing paranoid letters to the Duke of Edinburgh and Scotland Yard. In addition to being paranoid, she didn't care how she looked and her personal hygiene was poor. But after just two weeks of treatment with evening primrose oil and penicillin the woman began to lose her delusions. She improved so rapidly that after six weeks of treatment she looked at the paranoid letters she had written and said, amused, "I certainly wouldn't write such things now."

Another patient, a man, was first admitted to the hospital saying that he was Jesus Christ and that he had been talking to God. The doctors began treating him with penicillin and evening primrose oil, and his mental state improved after just one month. All aggressive behavior stopped after five months.

That the treatment worked in several months instead of years is remarkable, and shows the key role prostaglandin plays in treating this mental disorder.

VITAMINS FOR THERAPY

One theory holds that, in many cases, schizophrenia may be due to a person's abnormal metabolism of vitamins. According to Nobel-prize-winning scientist Linus Pauling, Ph.D., high-dosage vitamin therapy may be the key to avoiding thousands of hours of therapy for schizophrenia. Dr. Pauling and his associates studied the reactions of numerous schizophrenic patients to niacinamide and vitamins C and B_6. They found that 94 percent of diagnosed schizophrenics were low in at least one of the vitamins and that among the general population, those people who were low in all three vitamins were 40 times as likely to be hospitalized for schizophrenia sometime in their life.

Dr. Pauling's work is supported by a physician in the Philippines who uses large doses of B complex vitamins. Other nutrients are included, depending on the individual's case. This treatment is not widespread, but seems to be effective. One patient, a 26-year-old woman, had been schizophrenic for three years. She was irritable, violent, sharp tongued and refused to take baths. She spent most of her time lying down, but rarely slept. She improved after ten days, during which she was given oral supplements of a multi-vitamin, niacinamide, vitamin C and vitamin B_6. Two months later, the patient was reported to be greatly improved, with no more problems.

ELIMINATING GRAIN MAY HELP

It may be that a component of wheat leads to schizophrenia. Gluten, a

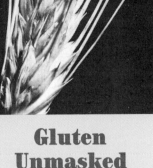

Gluten Unmasked

Gluten has long been thought to either cause or complicate schizophrenia. During World War II, when gluten-containing foods were rare in Greece, psychiatrists noted an improvement in the symptoms of schizophrenic patients. Numerous other studies also implicate gluten in schizophrenia.

Gluten is the protein that gives bread dough elasticity. It is found in large quantities in wheat. Barley, rye and oats can also cause problems.

No one knows exactly what in gluten causes problems, but some American researchers believe it may be substances called neuroactive peptides, which are formed in the body when gluten is digested.

Bright Light Conquers the Depression of Gloomy Days

Depressed? Feel like the gloomy world is closing in on you? Do you live your days as though you were shadowed by a dark cloud?

These images may be closer to reality than you think. Studies have shown that seasonal depression and anxiety in some people can be tied directly to the shorter days of winter. Dark days, it seems, can result in dark moods.

Researchers have labeled this winter depression SAD, for Seasonal Affective Disorder. Scientists at the National Institute of Mental Health (NIMH), in Bethesda, Maryland, believe that the so-called holiday blues, common at Christmas and the New Year, may often be due to dark days and long nights. That's probably why, say the researchers, most cultures brighten their December and January holidays with lights—like those on Christmas trees and in town squares.

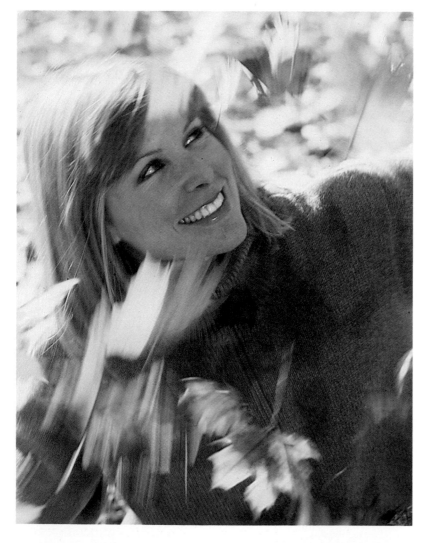

The NIMH researchers have been experimenting with artificial light as a treatment for this depression, with apparent success. They have been artificially lengthening the subjects' days by 3 hours in the morning and 3 in the evening. Their success has sparked other research into the effects of bright light on the gloom brought on by dark days.

This specific light comes from 8, 40-watt fluorescent "natural daylight" bulbs set in a light box. It's not a good idea to try the treatment at home, however. Instead, researchers advise that the long-term effects of the light therapy aren't known, and that sudden withdrawal from the treatment can result in severe emotional letdown. Another caution: Anyone with deep depression should be under professional care.

protein found in wheat, is thought to provoke the abnormal behavior of schizophrenia. A peculiar fact linking the disease to gluten is that it is extremely rare in countries where little or no gluten is ingested. For example, no schizophrenics were found in a 1947 survey of 1,955 people on Yap Island in Micronesia. But after 34 years of American influence, including a diet rich in wheat, there were 9.7 schizophrenics per 1,000 people.

This gluten connection was

brought home from the islands in a study of 16 schizophrenics conducted by researchers at the William S. Hall Psychiatric Institute in Columbia, South Carolina. The patients were studied while on a gluten-rich and then a gluten-free diet. While not all of the patients reacted to the changes in diet, a couple showed marked improvement. One woman who had been hospitalized for 13 years with a diagnosis of chronic schizophrenia had higher scores on mental evaluation tests after following a gluten-free diet. Her improvement was so dramatic, in fact, that her 13-year hospital ordeal ended and she returned home to live with her family.

Gluten is not the only substance that should be evaluated in any attempt to control schizophrenia. The coffee a schizophrenic drinks to clear his head may actually cloud it. Edwin J. Mikkelsen, M.D., of the National Institute of Mental Health in Bethesda, Maryland, has had several cases in which "caffeinism" aggravated schizophrenia. Dr. Mikkelson believes that caffeine aggravates the already abnormal nervous systems of schizophrenics, prompting the outbursts.

LIGHTING OUR DARKER MOODS

When someone totals the checkbook balance and then sighs, "I'm depressed," what they mean is that they are feeling unhappy. When you read that a famous person was hospitalized for severe depression, the condition described is quite different from unhappiness. Severe depression means withdrawal, loss of appetite, a profound sense of melancholia. Between the two conditions lies a wide range of emotion.

For the simple "blahs," doctors have found that a workout a day—or at least every other day—may take the blues away.

Regular physical activity may even keep them from coming around in the first place. "Exercise is emotional aerobics," says Bob Conroy, M.D., a psychiatrist at the Menninger Clinic in Topeka, Kansas, where he organized a cardiovascular fitness program that boosts sagging spirits.

"You don't have to run marathons, either, and we're not sold on just jogging. Any good aerobic routine [one that speeds up heart and breathing rates], carried on a minimum of three times a week for one hour each session, pays big dividends."

Run, dance, swim, play tennis or racquetball, take a brisk walk—there are many ways to work out your heart and soul.

If a solid hour of sustained exercise seems a bit too strenuous for you, don't despair. Other doctors have found that a more modest program also works to lift the spirits. "Just minor, nonvigorous exercise like walking a block can produce measurable, beneficial psychological changes," says Ronald Lawrence, M.D., Ph.D., a California psychiatrist and neurologist.

"It's estimated that one of every ten Americans suffers from depression," he says. "One thing that has made running in particular and exercise in general a success is that people can use it to treat their own depression."

Vitamins Counter Drug-Caused TD

People who are mentally ill and have depended on medication to control mental symptoms are at risk of developing tardive dyskinesia (TD)—uncontrollable muscle tics, spasms and speech disturbances. Often the disorder does *not* go away when the medication is stopped.

David Hawkins, M.D., and Charles Tkacz, M.D., directors of the North Nassau Mental Health Center in Manhasset, New York, have used nutritional therapy in combination with more traditional psychiatric methods. Along with antipsychotic drugs, they have been using vitamins C, E, B_6 and niacin or niacinamide to treat schizophrenia and other disorders.

During the summer of 1978, although reports of TD were appearing with alarming frequency, they found "to our astonishment that among our patient population (10,000 outpatients during a 10-year period; 1,000 inpatients at our hospital during a 10-year period) *not one case* of tardive dyskinesia developed."

One way exercise may do this is by increasing the levels of serotonin, a neurotransmitter in the brain. Scientists have found that levels of serotonin are lower in people who are seriously depressed, and that a jump

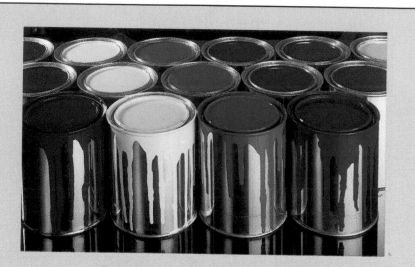

Getting the Lead Out

Mental retardation is a tragedy affecting the whole family. A retarded child requires near-constant attention and guidance. Many times, the retardation is caused by physical injury or an unavoidable birth defect. But one cause of this dreadful condition is preventable: lead poisoning.

Lead is all around us. Because of industrial and automobile pollution, it has become a part of the air, earth, food and water. Scottish scientists studied the homes of retarded children and found that the children drank and bathed in water that contained much higher levels of lead than water available in the homes of normal children.

The lead can come directly from the environment, from chips of old paint or even from the mother before birth. But there are ways to keep lead away from your child. Use distilled water for drinking and formula preparation. Also be sure the diets of older children include calcium, vitamin D and zinc. All help prevent lead from building up in the body. And encourage children to exercise, as well. It seems that regular exercise—such as running 10 miles a week—causes the body to better metabolize calcium. And when calcium is handled better, so is lead, which follows the same metabolic process. The end result is that exercisers excrete more lead.

in serotonin levels goes hand in hand with feeling better mentally.

Another way to raise serotonin levels is to increase your intake of the amino acid tryptophan. In one study, researchers compared tryptophan with an antidepressant drug called amitriptyline. The drug is very effective in relieving the symptoms of depression, but it can be toxic and leaves severe side effects in its wake. Tryptophan, on the other hand, is virtually harmless. Very few users suffer even mild side effects, and those who do report that the side effects are transient.

The study, which took about 12 weeks, tested a group of 115 patients who were divided into four study groups. One group took only tryptophan, another took only amitriptyline, a third group took a combination of the two and a control group took a placebo, a harmless but ineffective "dummy" medication.

At the end of the experiment, the researchers found that tryptophan was just as effective in relieving depression as the antidepressant medication. And tryptophan offers the enormous benefit of being rapidly metabolized and safe.

SAFE, DRUG-FREE CONTROL OF MANIA

Another use for tryptophan is in the treatment of mania—a sporadic mental disorder characterized by rapid talking, exaggerated emotions and hyperactive movements. Guy Chouinard, M.D., of McGill University in Montreal, says that tryptophan is an effective mood stabilizer. He gave it to 24 mania patients for one week, and the mental state of 14 patients improved. During the second week, half the group continued to take tryptophan and half were given a placebo. Eight of the tryptophan patients improved but 4 worsened. But among the group receiving a placebo, only 1 improved, while 6 were unchanged and 5 got worse.

Lecithin also may work wonders for people suffering with mania. Patients given lecithin by New England researchers showed measurable improvement. The patients recovered so quickly that they were able to leave the hospital after just 3½ weeks instead of the usual 8 weeks. "Lithium has been used as the drug to treat mania and it has been effective in 80 percent of the cases," said one of the researchers. "The problem is it's only a treatment and not a cure. So, we're looking for a cure. And that's why we're looking at lecithin."

THEY HELPED THEMSELVES AND BEAT AUTISM

Autistic children look normal, and can be expected to live out a normal life span, but they have serious difficulties socializing, learning and communicating. They aren't just withdrawn; they seem totally removed from the normal realm of human activity. Autistics can have IQ's ranging from low to high. Regardless of intelligence level, however, comprehension is erratic. For example, a child might be able to learn to walk but be unable to comprehend toilet training. Autism is more common in boys than in girls, and it does not appear to be an inherited disease.

One lucky child is Raun Kaufman, who at age one was diagnosed as being autistic. Fortunately, his parents didn't just despair at the diagnosis. They worked around the clock to help Raun cross the bridge from his imaginary world to their reality.

First they read all they could about the disease and spoke to several doctors. No one offered them much hope for Raun. So they set out on their own to help their child. The first step was to accept Raun for what he was, without judgment. If Raun sat on the floor spinning plates around and around, his family would join in. They wanted him to feel approval for each thing he did.

The second step was to motivate Raun to leave his shell, by making him realize the world was beautiful and exciting. After weeks spent in long days of stimulation with music, food and movement, Raun attempted to communicate with people.

Bad Mix: Aspirin, Fevers, Children

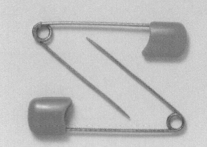

Parents shouldn't automatically reach for the aspirin when their children develop a fever—especially if the fever is the result of a viral infection like chicken pox or influenza. Several studies have linked aspirin used to treat viral infections to Reye's syndrome, a life-threatening childhood disease that can cause seizures, fast breathing and coma. According to Samuel Gotoff, M.D., of Michael Reese Hospital in Chicago, "Children tolerate fevers better than adults do." Although parents may want to call the doctor, they needn't be alarmed unless the fever rises above 104 degrees, because, says Dr. Gotoff, "fever is nature's way to fight infections."

Meanwhile, parents can lower the fever by giving acetaminophen (e.g., Tylenol) and making certain the child drinks extra liquids, instead of using aspirin.

After reading about studies done with disturbed children and food additives, the Kaufmans looked at the labels on the products on their kitchen shelves and realized that they "read like the Who's Who list in chemistry." They ditched the chemicals for organic, mostly unprocessed foods, and dropped red meat from the family diet.

After 30 weeks of attention, stimulation, a teaching program and a good diet of healthy, chemical-free foods, Raun was talking and showed a great awareness of the world around him. The Kaufmans took Raun back to the institution where he had been rediagnosed as autistic just four months before. Tests were done, and to the doctors' surprise (but not the persevering Kaufmans') Raun was functioning at his normal age level. A happy ending.

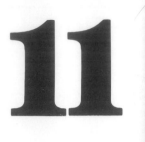

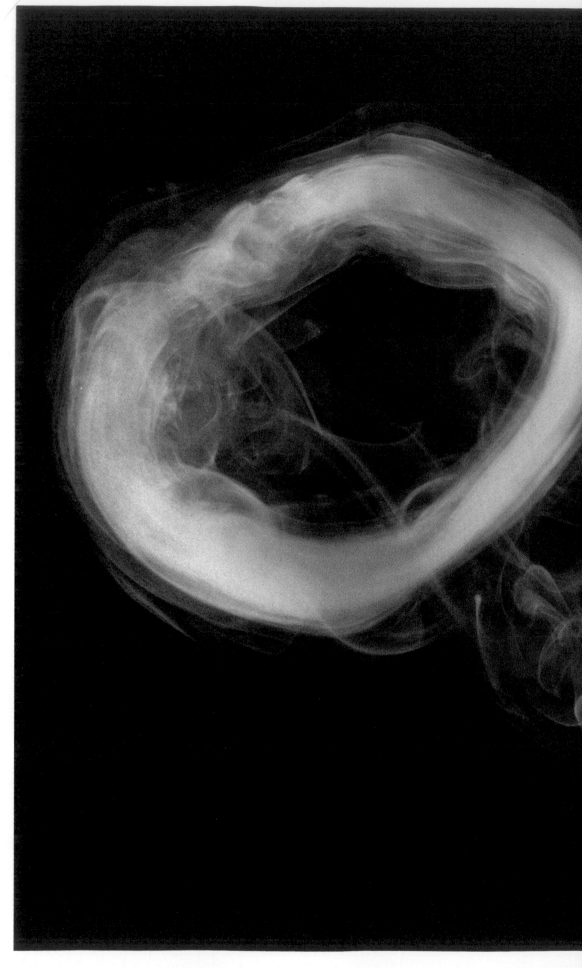

Freedom from Addictions

Not "bad habits," addictions
are real illnesses that can be
treated and often cured.

Addiction is a misunderstood illness. Consider this: Someone addicted to heroin, for example, is thought to be a threat to the community, while someone equally hooked, but instead hooked on nicotine, still can be seen as an upstanding citizen. Heavy drinking is sometimes considered a weakness, sometimes a disease—but smoking marijuana is often not considered at all. Its use has become so common that it no longer raises eyebrows, not even the eyebrows under a police cap. And somehow "to snort" has become a chic verb, but only when it precedes the noun "cocaine."

Most people have used one or more of these drugs. But how can you tell if you or someone you care about is *addicted?* Generally speaking, drug use is neither recreational nor therapeutic if you: find you need larger amounts to get the same effect; depend on the drug physically or psychologically and suffer withdrawal symptoms if you go without; spend a lot of time thinking about how to get it and when to use it. In other words, when the drug controls you, you're addicted.

Addiction harms the body as much as diabetes or any other long-term, debilitating disease. In fact, the newest medical thinking says that addiction *is* a physical illness—not a crime or a mental aberration. Unfortunately, medical science usually has only one way of responding to illness: Prescribe a drug. And so the "treatment" for addiction often consists of substituting one harmful (and sometimes equally addictive) drug for another. Thus, a person isn't a heroin addict stealing TV's to support his habit; he's hooked on methadone that's given out free at a clinic. Or the cigarette smoker chews on nicotine gum. In short, the addict is still an addict—only now he's using a more socially acceptable and perhaps slightly less toxic drug.

But the revolution in medical thought that's responsible for now regarding addiction as a physical illness has also produced a revolution in treatment. Some very encouraging research, discussed here in detail, shows how nutrition, exercise and other natural methods can heal the addicted body *and* reduce the cravings that make addiction such torture—thus stopping addiction once and for all.

THE BUTT STOPS HERE

Chances are you already know that cigarettes cause lung cancer. But did you know that smoking is the most important cause of the respiratory diseases emphysema and bronchitis, and an important contributor to asthma, influenza and respiratory infections?

Aside from breathing disorders, smoking also contributes to hardening of the arteries, high blood pressure, stroke and bone loss, and it can cause gastrointestinal problems, including ulcers.

If you think switching to low-tar, low-nicotine cigarettes is the answer, you're only fooling yourself.

Smokers of so-called "low-yield" cigarettes do not consume any less nicotine than smokers of regular cigarettes, according to a study of people who smoked 15 brands of commercial cigarettes. The researchers say that's because manufacturers cite nicotine yields produced by smoking machines, not by people—who take deeper, more frequent puffs. Other studies have shown that low-tar, low-nicotine cigarettes produce just as much carbon monoxide as regular cigarettes do, if not more. So there's no such thing as a "safe" cigarette.

A DIET TO HELP YOU QUIT PAINLESSLY

Certainly quitting cigarettes is easier said than done. Nicotine is a powerful—and versatile—drug. It can give you a lift, calm you down, keep you company when you're bored, comfort you in times of stress.

Okay, so you enjoy smoking but wish you didn't. Chances are you've tried to quit—more than once. (The success rate is less than 25 percent.) Clearly, something is being overlooked.

That "something" may be a little-known effect of nicotine on body chemistry. A small number of doctors have discovered that the real reason people have such a tough time unshackling themselves from cigarettes may be nicotine's ability to acidify the body.

The theory germinated when Stanley Schacter, Ph.D., a professor of psychology at Columbia University, found that people with highly acidic urine generally smoke more than those with alkaline urine. Dr. Schacter and his associates also noted that nine out of ten smokers had distinctly more acidic urine on stressful days. And they craved cigarettes more intensely on more stressful days.

Dr. Schacter theorized that perhaps this acidity caused people to smoke more. What's more, he found that acid urine rapidly eliminates nicotine from the body. To replace it, smokers tend to smoke more.

The link between smoking and body chemistry was then pursued by A. James Fix, Ph.D., and David M.

When You Quit Smoking, Benefits Begin Immediately

Suppose you quit smoking now, right this instant. Surprisingly, your health would begin to improve almost at once, and soon you'd be able to once again smell the flowers.

- In 9 hours, your blood pressure, if elevated, would begin to return to normal.
- Within 12 hours, levels of nicotine and carbon monoxide in your blood would fall, and your heart and lungs would begin to heal.
- Within just a few days, you'd regain your lost senses of taste and smell, breathe more easily and feel stronger, clearheaded and energetic.

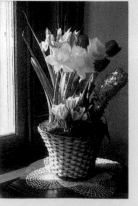

Daughton, two behavioral researchers at the University of Nebraska College of Medicine. To make a long story short, Dr. Fix and his colleague came up with a diet that discourages the craving for cigarettes by alkalizing body chemistry—specifically the urine. The diet emphasizes vegetables (which create an alkaline urine) and downplays meat or cheese (which have an acidic effect). The diet focuses on foods that cut the nicotine craving most, such as molasses, dried beans, raisins, figs, beet greens, spinach, brewer's yeast, almonds and carrots. It includes, to a lesser extent, soybean flour, celery, grapefruit, white and sweet potatoes, dried peas, tomatoes, strawberries and bananas. Smokers should avoid wheat germ, lentils, macaroni or spaghetti, chicken, eggs, steak, liver, lamb chops, codfish and cheese— they acidify the urine.

Speaking of diet, one of the main reasons people resist trying to quit cigarettes is the fear of gaining weight. They've heard of former smokers who "automatically" gained 10 to 15 pounds and never could shed them.

"There is a theory that says that when you smoke, your metabolism speeds up and when you quit, it slows down, causing weight gain," says Judith K. Ockene, Ph.D., who's written extensively on smoking behavior. "But just as likely a reason that smokers gain weight after they quit is because they eat more. They begin to use food in the same way that they used cigarettes—to relieve anxiety, to deal with anger, depression or stress, or simply out of boredom."

ALCOHOLISM: A NO-FAULT DISEASE

Ever wonder why the synonym for "drunk" is "intoxicated"? The key part of that word, toxic, explains the connection. When you drink, the body breaks down alcohol into various toxic substances—substances that can result in liver damage, pancreatic damage and more. Large amounts of alcohol may increase blood fats and contribute to heart disease. Around 50 percent of all alcoholics have high blood pressure, which can lead to strokes. A study of 172 stroke victims showed that 22 percent had been drinking within 24 hours of the stroke.

Alcoholics can't sleep well or think quickly. Moreover, in many cases they have the recall of people who are years older. No wonder: Autopsies have shown that the brains of alcoholics actually shrink.

With prolonged heavy drinking, sexual urge dwindles. So does performance. And all that occurs in addition to the heavy toll alcoholism takes on one's personal, professional and family life.

Yet alcoholism is no more your fault than is, say, diabetes. And you can no more talk yourself out of this disease than you can talk yourself out of having diabetes or any other serious disorder. The latest evidence traces alcohol dependence to abnormalities in the way certain people

At about a dollar a pack, the money spent on cigarettes in a year really adds up. Stashed in a "ciggybank," instead of going up in smoke, that money might buy a Caribbean vacation, some fabulous clothes or a stereo system—depending on how much you customarily smoke. (If you put the money in a savings account, where it can earn interest, you could amass even more!)

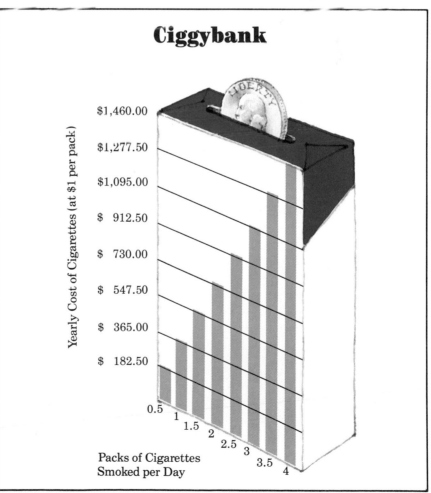

Ciggybank

Yearly Cost of Cigarettes (at $1 per pack)

$1,460.00
$1,277.50
$1,095.00
$ 912.50
$ 730.00
$ 547.50
$ 365.00
$ 182.50

0.5 1 1.5 2 2.5 3 3.5 4

Packs of Cigarettes Smoked per Day

break it down (metabolize it). Experts in the study of alcoholism compared blood samples taken from male alcoholics and nonalcoholics. What they found is that the alcoholics' blood contained a specific compound *not* found in the blood of nonalcoholics. Its presence indicated a defect in alcohol metabolism.

Other research contributes to the theory that alcoholism is a physical disease, not a mental disorder. Joan Mathews-Larson, director of Health Recovery Center, a drug and alcoholism treatment clinic in Minneapolis, feels that because of whatever genetic defect alcoholics share, they react to alcohol in a biochemically different manner than do nonalcoholics. And if alcoholism is the result of a biochemical defect, it can be treated by changing the chemistry of the body—with nutrition.

NUTRITION: A BETTER WAY TO FIGHT ALCOHOLISM

Alcoholics are among the most malnourished people in the world, even if they eat well (and they often don't). Because of damage to the liver, stomach and other digestive organs, alcoholics don't absorb or utilize vitamins, and they excrete many minerals—leaving shortages of nearly all essential nutrients.

Many doctors ignore all but a few frank nutrient deficiencies and concentrate primarily on treating the psychological side of alcoholism. With "talk therapy," only about one-third of all dried-out alcoholics don't go back to drinking. But when nutritional therapy is added, the success rate skyrockets.

Nutrition, in fact, may be the key to treating many aspects of this addiction, as well as treating alcoholism as a whole. We know, for example, that alcoholism can lead to deficiencies of vitamin A and zinc, because of damage to the liver (a primary site of alcohol metabolism). Replacing vitamin A can help to correct ailing night vision, so common among this group.

According to Roger Williams, Ph.D., further supplements of all the B vitamins can reduce the craving for alcohol. Moreover, Dr. Williams also has recommended glutamine, an amino acid. He began giving glutamine to alcoholics over 25 years ago, to break their insatiable craving for alcohol.

To supply an alcoholic's special needs for various nutrients, Dr. Williams also formulated a regimen that includes:

Vitamins. Vitamin A, 7,500 I.U.; vitamin D, 400 I.U.; vitamin E, 40 I.U.; vitamin C, 250 milligrams; thiamine, 2 milligrams; riboflavin, 2 milligrams; vitamin B_6, 3 milligrams;

Alcohol is the major cause of accidents of all kinds, according to a report by Kimball I. Maull, M.D., of the division of trauma at the Medical College of Virginia in Richmond. Alcohol is not only responsible for half of all fatal auto crashes, but drinking is also to blame for many home accidents and more than half of all fatal falls, choking deaths, drownings, burns and assaults. That's because alcohol interferes with judgment, impairs perception and coordination and sparks aggression and violence in many people. What's more, a person is likely to injure himself more seriously when alcohol is involved than when it is not.

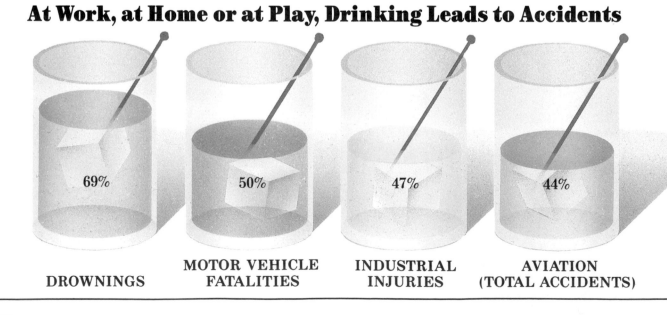

At Work, at Home or at Play, Drinking Leads to Accidents

| 69% | 50% | 47% | 44% |
| DROWNINGS | MOTOR VEHICLE FATALITIES | INDUSTRIAL INJURIES | AVIATION (TOTAL ACCIDENTS) |

vitamin B$_{12}$, 9 micrograms; niacinamide, 20 milligrams; pantothenate, 15 milligrams; biotin, 0.3 milligrams; folate, 0.4 milligrams; choline, 250 milligrams; inositol, 250 milligrams; para-aminobenzoic acid, 30 milligrams; and rutin, 200 milligrams.

Minerals. Calcium, 250 milligrams; magnesium, 200 milligrams; iron, 5 milligrams; zinc, 15 milligrams, chromium, 1 milligram; and selenium, 0.05 milligrams. (This nutritional program should be followed only under a doctor's supervision.)

Nutritionist Lillian Yung, Ed.D., studied a group of 64 alcoholics to see whether those who stayed sober ate differently than those who went back to the bottle. She found that 45 percent of the people who stayed sober for more than 50 days after leaving treatment used vitamin supplements. Only 19 percent of those who went back to the bottle used supplements. Clearly, nutrition can make the difference in how well you do.

Other doctors are equally enthusiastic about the nutritional approach. Mixing vitamins and psychotherapy has helped many alcoholics turn their lives around in a few months, says Harry K. Panjwani, M.D., a former member of the advisory committee of the National Council on Alcoholism. Dr. Panjwani puts each new patient

on glutamine, niacinamide and vitamin C—at least 500 milligrams of each every day.

The dual approach is very encouraging, especially when you consider that until recently, the *only* hope a recovering alcoholic had was the support of groups like Alcoholics Anonymous (AA).

"In many AA meetings, people unknowingly do things that impede their recovery—drinking coffee, smoking cigarettes and eating sweets," says Ms. Mathews-Larson. "Most AA people aren't aware of the biochemical nature of alcoholism. And you can't 'talk away' alcoholism's effects."

SMOOTH THE PEAKS AND VALLEYS— WITHOUT TRANQUILIZERS

One of the most widely prescribed drugs in the United States is not aspirin, penicillin or the birth control pill, but Valium. In fact, millions of American adults often use a tranquilizer of some kind.

"Valium has been prescribed for everything from dandruff to ingrown toenails," says Conway Hunter Jr., M.D., former medical director of the Addictive Disease Unit, Peachford Hospital, Atlanta, Georgia. "And it works. Because if you take enough Valium, you don't care about the prob-

"Gusto" Ads Hype Booze

Advertisements featuring athletes and other celebrities hawking beer, wine and liquor glamorize drinking. They link alcohol with sexual, social and business success. Moreover, they tout alcohol as a grand reward for a job well done.

Critics say such advertising encourages alcohol abuse. They believe equal time should be given to ads that show that it's okay *not* to drink. After all, if you only go 'round once in life, it might help to be sober.

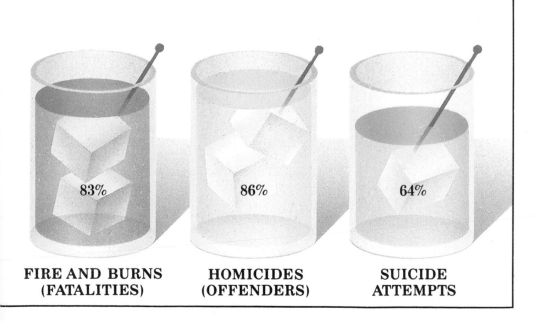

FIRE AND BURNS (FATALITIES)   83%

HOMICIDES (OFFENDERS)   86%

SUICIDE ATTEMPTS   64%

lem. But it's *extremely* dangerous."

Valium doesn't just calm you down—it knocks you out. In one study, 40 elderly men who took the drug became tired, forgetful and clumsy. That makes taking Valium just as risky as drinking alcohol if you have to drive a car or operate machinery.

What's more, tranquilizers can cause brain damage. When doctors tested the brain function of 66 heavy users of sedatives, nearly half were mildly to moderately impaired.

Tranquilizers are used to calm a person without causing drowsiness. They include diazepam (Valium), chlordiazepoxide (Librium), oxazepam (Serax), clorazepate dipotassium (Tranxene), halazepam (Paxipam), prazepam (Centrax) and lorazepam (Ativan). People begin to take these drugs primarily—but not exclusively —to relieve anxiety, tension and sleeplessness.

Ironically, sleeping pills (a type of tranquilizer) can cause some of the very problems they're supposed to treat. An editorial in *Lancet* says that sleeping pills have "the effect of hampering natural sleep when the drug is stopped—indeed, anxiety may be increased. The consequent insomnia, restlessness and night-mares lead to a request for repetition of the prescription, and dependence is thus established." You're left with your original insomnia—*plus* a drug habit.

Make no mistake about it—tranquilizers are addictive in the truest sense of the word. Withdrawal may involve any of a host of symptoms, from nausea and dizziness to skin rashes and convulsions. And withdrawal can last *years,* says Dr. Hunter.

"Withdrawal may not begin until ten days or later after you stop taking Valium," says Dr. Hunter. "First you go through a brief period of discomfort. But six weeks later, your whole world turns topsy-turvy, with possible convulsions, burning skin rashes, any of a whole list of problems that neither you nor your doctor relate to the drug you stopped taking weeks earlier. So you may be put back on Valium. It's a vicious cycle."

To get free of tranquilizers, you can't quit cold turkey. To ease withdrawal, you need to taper the dosage. And you need to replace the tranquilizer with a positive lifestyle, including relaxation techniques, proper nutrition and exercise, says Dr. Hunter. He also suggests that people who want to stop taking tranquilizers seek medical help from a doctor who knows what to expect. Otherwise, withdrawal can be brutal.

Let's expand Dr. Hunter's techniques with specific suggestions:

Sexism and Tranquilizers: Women's Ills Are "All in the Head"

If men and women approach a doctor for treatment of an infection, either sex is likely to receive antibiotics. However, for less clear-cut health problems, women are given tranquilizers more often than men are.

ANTIBIOTICS PRESCRIBED

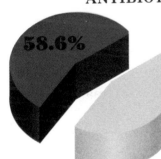

For Women
(age 25-44)

58.6%

For Men
(age 25-44)

41.3%

TRANQUILIZERS PRESCRIBED

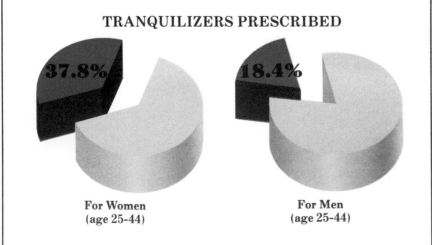

For Women
(age 25-44)

37.8%

For Men
(age 25-44)

18.4%

Meditation and Other Relaxation Techniques. People who meditate report an increased feeling of self-worth and a reduction of fear, envy and jealousy—positive changes that help to give them the strength to get along without tranquilizers. Meditation also appears to lower blood lactate, a by-product of muscle metabolism. High levels of lactate have been associated with irritability and anxiety attacks.

To meditate, simply take off your shoes, sit comfortably in a quiet room and close your eyes. Take three or four deep breaths. Relax all your muscles from feet to head. For 10 minutes, repeat to yourself a simple word or syllable with each exhalation of breath. Ignore all extraneous thoughts and sounds. Then open your eyes and think about how relaxed you feel.

Imagery. To help your body recover from tranquilizer use, Dr. Hunter recommends positive imagery. For example, imagine you are lying on a rubber raft, drifting on a tranquil pond, with the warm morning sun relaxing every muscle. Feel the tension disappear and your mind clear.

Exercise. Lack of exercise is a common cause of anxiety and insomnia, which in turn are major reasons that people use tranquilizers. Regular, vigorous physical activity can dispel a lot of tension and relieve insomnia without tranquilizers. For example, researchers at Stanford University School of Medicine tested 81 sedentary men. Those who ran regularly during a year's time showed significantly less anxiety than nonrunners in the group.

"Running, dance, yoga, hiking, swimming and just simple walking are potent antianxiety agents," says Harold H. Bloomfield, M.D., a San Diego psychiatrist.

The Serenity Vitamins. A case of "nerves" can be triggered by poor diet. On top of that, anxiety and stressful situations can increase the need for certain nutrients—beginning with the B vitamins.

"I recommend large amounts of the B vitamins, particularly niacin," says Dr. Hunter. "Niacin smooths the peaks and valleys, restores the normal balance of elation and deflation. [Generally, people shouldn't take more than 50 milligrams of any B vitamin on their own.]

"I also recommend vitamin E, particularly for women, because it regulates the effect of hormones," says Dr. Hunter. "And I recommend that people avoid sugar and lower their intake of overly refined carbohydrates."

If you're a woman and your nerves act up before your menstrual period, try extra vitamin B_6. In one experiment, conducted by Joel T. Hargrove, M.D., and Guy E. Abraham, M.D., 25 women suffering from moderate to severe premenstrual tension were given either vitamin B_6 or a placebo.

At the end of the study the doctors found that 21 out of 25 suffered fewer or less severe symptoms when they took the B_6, but not when they took the placebo. Some doctors who give B_6 for premenstrual tension recommend beginning with 50 milligrams a day.

Soothing Beverages. Caffeine can make you hyper and alcohol can interfere with sleep. Instead, switch to herb tea, fruit or vegetable juices, seltzer water or club soda with lemon juice, or other nonstimulating beverages.

Support Groups. "Organizations such as Narcotics Anonymous exist in nearly every community and can be extremely helpful," says Dr. Hunter. "They're one of the most therapeutic methods a person can use to weather withdrawal. All these steps create a positive lifestyle, which works for dependencies of many types."

MARIJUANA: WHY THEY CALL IT "DOPE"

Despite its increasing social acceptance, marijuana is, nevertheless, a dangerous drug.

Smoking one joint punishes the lungs with as much tar as ten medium-tar cigarettes, according to research done at the University of

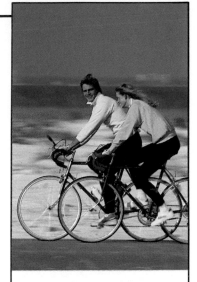

Tranquillity and Peace— Without Drugs

Nervous? You can tame anxiety, insomnia and depression with:

- Exercise
- Meditation
- B vitamins and calcium
- Deep breathing
- Imagery
- Serene music
- Soothing beverages

California School of Public Health in Berkeley. Marijuana smoke contains 50 percent more cancer-causing hydrocarbons than cigarette smoke. Altogether, marijuana may have the same potential for causing cancer as cigarettes. In fact, regular marijuana smokers often develop a chronic dry cough that sounds a lot like the cough of someone who smokes cigarettes. Donald Taskin, M.D., a lung specialist at UCLA, found that

people who smoked an average of five joints a week for at least two years had worse lung function than people the same age who smoked 16 or more cigarettes a day.

Those and countless other studies have been compiled by the Institute of Medicine in a 188-page report called *Marijuana and Health*. Here are a few highlights:

- Marijuana stresses the circulation by increasing heart rate and sometimes blood pressure.
- In males, marijuana causes decreased movement of sperm and lowers sperm count and levels of testosterone (the principal male hormone)—in effect, making men less virile.
- In females, marijuana may interfere with ovulation, causing temporary infertility, and may increase the risk of miscarriage.
- Chronic use also impairs memory and slows learning.
- Driving when you're high is as dangerous as driving when you're drunk.

Young people often try marijuana for the same reason they smoke cigarettes or drink alcohol—peer pressure. Recent figures show that up to 50 percent of all high school students have smoked pot. What are the telltale signs that point to a possible problem?

- An abrupt change in general mood or attitude.
- A sudden decline in attendance or performance at school or work.
- A sudden resistance to discipline.
- Increased borrowing of money, or stealing.
- Heightened secrecy about activities.
- Association with friends who use drugs.

The most effective way to convince kids that they shouldn't smoke pot is to present them with the facts. The medical evidence of marijuana's harmful effects on the lungs, brain, heart and reproductive performance makes getting high lose much of its appeal. Surveys show that when kids do quit, it's because they're worried about physical and psychological damage, including loss of energy or ambition.

Pot Targets the Brain

Smoking marijuana makes you high, but not without a price. THC (the active ingredient in marijuana) travels to the brain, where it triggers subtle changes in brain chemistry that affect mental function and behavior. Getting high on pot slows learning, impairs memory, muddles your thinking and understanding and generally makes you dumber than you should be. Moreover, smoking cannabis can produce anxiety, confusion and disorientation—in effect, putting you in a temporary state of senility.

Contrary to popular belief, smoking marijuana does not liberate your personality and enhance personal relationships. Instead, you become insecure and rather detached.

All in all, smoking marijuana makes you a lesser person than you really are.

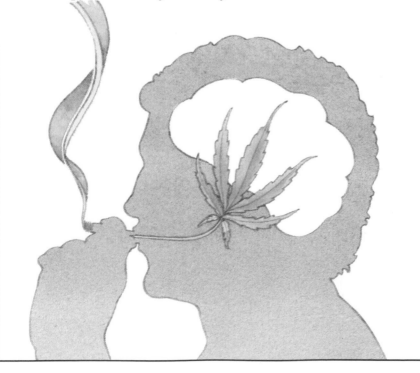

COCAINE: COSTLY IN MORE WAYS THAN ONE

Some say there's no kick like cocaine. Why else would anyone spend a month's salary for brief flashes of euphoria?

The high cost, however, isn't the only problem with cocaine. First of all, the rumors you may have heard about addicts having their noses rebuilt are true. Repeated snorting irritates the mucous lining of the nose and eventually wears a hole in the septum (the partition between the nostrils). Yet people continue to indulge, even after surgery.

Not all coke damage is so easily repaired. Two researchers exposed rats to cocaine and found that in the nasal passage it metabolized into formaldehyde—a chemical that may cause nasal cancer.

Cocaine also can cause fatal heart attacks—even in healthy young adults. A 38-year-old man developed angina and eventually suffered a heart attack after snorting cocaine, according to doctors at the department of medicine, University of California, San Francisco. In fact, a number of doctors have reported assorted cardiovascular reactions to cocaine, including rapid or irregular heartbeat, high blood pressure—and death.

When people decide to kick the cocaine habit, it's usually not out of concern for their health, but because it ruins the quality of their lives.

"Coke becomes an obsession," says Joan Mathews-Larson of the Health Recovery Center in Minneapolis. "Users spend more than they earn and will ransom anything of value to get more cocaine. People think they'll never reach that point, but they often do."

Coke is *very* addictive, psychologically. "Because cocaine can make people feel so good for so short a time—and not so good immediately afterward—people tend to go on using it, trying to get back the good feeling," says Andrew Weil, M.D., who's studied addictive disease extensively.

"Anything that takes you that high brings you pretty far down," says Ms. Mathews-Larson. "When you're not high, you don't feel normal, you feel *terrible*." Withdrawal leaves you melancholy, sluggish, jittery and unhappy.

"How successfully coke addicts kick the habit depends on how actively they pursue a new lifestyle—exercise, nutrition, relaxation," she says. "Exercise is vital because coke users need to replace the drug with something that energizes the body and gives them a lift for the energy they need.

"They also need a crash program of nutrition. Vitamin C and B complex deficiencies are common among cocaine addicts. At the clinic, we start them on large doses, because nutritional status is usually poor in the beginning. But then we cut the dosage back as they improve," says Ms. Mathews-Larson.

In addition to good nutrition, stress management also helps lick the problem.

Dr. Conway Hunter says, "I recommend a lot of vigorous physical activity—especially aerobics—coupled with mental and spiritual techniques, including relaxation. They're good for all of us, but they're especially good for people with a dependency, because they improve self-worth and confidence."

Vitamin C and Heroin Addiction

Vitamin C may ease withdrawal from heroin and can reduce craving for the drug, according to Alfred F. Libby, Ph.D., director of a drug abuse treatment center in San Clemente, California.

Apparently, heroin addiction creates a chronic deficiency of vitamin C, among other nutrients. Individuals undergoing detoxification are tested and given massive amounts of vitamin C intravenously, plus custom-tailored amounts of all the B vitamins, calcium, magnesium and a special formula of amino acids.

By decontaminating the body of all traces of heroin toxins, the vitamin C-centered approach reduces the craving for heroin, breaking the addiction. Best of all, no withdrawal symptoms occur—no diarrhea, vomiting, runny nose, muscle spasms or convulsions. In his most recent study, done at an acute care hospital, Dr. Libby treated 11 heroin addicts with this method. All remained drug free for 14 months or longer.

Source Notes

Chapter 1
Page 7

"Food Sources of Potassium" adapted from *Nutritive Value of American Foods in Common Units*, Agriculture Handbook No. 456, by Catherine F. Adams (Washington, D.C.: Agricultural Research Service, U.S. Department of Agriculture, 1975)
and
Composition of Foods: Dairy and Egg Products, Agriculture Handbook No. 8-1, by Consumer and Food Economics Institute (Washington, D.C.: Agricultural Research Service, U.S. Department of Agriculture, 1976)
and
Composition of Foods: Fruit and Fruit Juices, Agriculture Handbook No. 8-9, by Consumer Nutrition Center (Washington, D.C.: Human Nutrition Information Service, U.S. Department of Agriculture, 1982)
and
Composition of Foods: Poultry Products, Agriculture Handbook No. 8-5, by Consumer and Food Economics Institute (Washington, D.C.: Science and Education Administration, U.S. Department of Agriculture, 1979).

Chapter 2
Page 20

"Pollen Concentrations in the United States" adapted from "Respiratory Atopic Disease," by Kenneth P. Mathews, M.D., *Journal of the American Medical Association*, November 26, 1982. Copyright 1982 by the American Medical Association. Reprinted by permission of the publisher and author.

Chapter 5
Page 79

"High-Fiber Disease Fighters" adapted from *McCance and Widdowson's The Composition of Foods*, by A. A. Paul and D. A. T. Southgate (New York: Elsevier/North Holland Biomedical Press, 1978)
and
Nutritive Value of American Foods in Common Units, Agriculture Handbook No. 456, by Catherine F. Adams (Washington, D.C.: Agricultural Research Service, U.S. Department of Agriculture, 1975)
and
"Composition of Foods Commonly Used in Diets for Persons with Diabetes," by James W. Anderson, Wen-Ju Lin and Kyleen Ward, *Diabetes Care*, September/October 1978
and
Composition of Foods: Soups, Sauces and Gravies, Agriculture Handbook No. 8-6, by Consumer and Food Economics Institute (Washington, D.C.: Science and Education Administration, U.S. Department of Agriculture, 1980)
and
Composition of Foods: Spices and Herbs, Agriculture Handbook No. 8-2, by Consumer and Food Economics Institute (Washington, D.C.: Agricultural Research Service, U.S. Department of Agriculture, 1977)
and
"Topics in Dietary Fiber" and "Fiber Analysis Tables," Reports of Research of the Cornell University Agricultural Experiment Station, 1978
and
Information supplied by cereal companies.

Chapter 6
Page 88

"Once Again, Breast Is Best" adapted from "Childhood Celiac Disease is Disappearing," by J. M. Littlewood, Avril J. Crollick and I. D. G. Richards, *Lancet*, December 20/27, 1980.

Page 90

"Incidence of Ulcerative Colitis" adapted from "Incidence Rates of Ulcerative Colitis and Crohn's Disease in Fifteen Areas of the United States," by Cedric F. Garland, et al, *Gastroenterology*, vol. 81. Copyright 1981 by The American Gastroenterological Association. Reprinted by permission of the publisher.

Chapter 7
Page 107

"Blood Sugar of Diabetics on Low- and High-Fiber Diets" adapted from *Diabetes: A Practical New Guide to Healthy Living*, by James W. Anderson (New York: Arco Publishing, 1981).

Chapter 9
Page 132

"The Plummeting Sperm Count" adapted from "Singular Trends in Reported Sperm Counts," by W. H. James, *Andrologia*, vol. 12, no. 4, 1980.

Chapter 10
Page 138

"Cigarette Smoke Can Cloud Hearing" adapted from "Cigarette Smoking and Hearing Loss," by Amal S. Ibrahim and Ahmed S. Fatthi, *World Smoking and Health*, Summer 1982.

Page 147

"Food Sources of Manganese" adapted from *Nutritive Value of American Foods in Common Units*, Agriculture Handbook No. 456, by Catherine F. Adams (Washington, D.C.: Agricultural Research Service, U.S. Department of Agriculture, 1975)
and
Composition of Foods: Breakfast Cereals, Agriculture Handbook No. 8-8, by Consumer Nutrition Center (Washington, D.C., Human Nutrition Information Service, U.S. Department of Agriculture, 1982)
and
Composition of Foods: Fruits and Fruit Juices, Agriculture Handbook No. 8-9, by Consumer Nutrition Center (Washington, D.C.: Human Nutrition Information Service, U.S. Department of Agriculture, 1982)
and
Composition of Foods: Poultry Products, Agriculture Handbook No. 8-5, by Consumer and Food Economics Institute (Washington, D.C.: Science and Education Administration, U.S. Department of Agriculture, 1979).

Chapter 11
Pages 158-159

"At Work, at Home or at Play, Drinking Leads to Accidents" adapted from the Third Special Report to Congress on Alcohol and Health, Ernest P. Noble, ed. (Rockville, Md.: National Institute for Alcohol Abuse and Alcoholism, 1978).

Page 160

"Sexism and Tranquilizers: Women's Ills Are All in the Head" adapted from "Prescribing Tranquilizers to Women and Men," by John E. Anderson, *CMA Journal*, December 1981.

Photography Credits

Cover: John Hamel.
Staff Photographers—
Angelo M. Caggiano: pp.
10, bottom right; 21; 29;
72; 82; 91; 118; 147. Carl
Doney: pp. 15; 32-33; 107;
112-113. T. L. Gettings:
pp. 24; 60; 97; 130.
John P. Hamel: pp. 149;
154-155. Mitchell T.
Mandel: pp. viii-1; 10-11;
41; 52-53; 68-69; 134-135;
141. Alison Miksch:
pp. 35; 45; 64; 66-67; 78;
93; 108; 153. Anthony
Rodale: pp. 83; 121. Pat
Seip: p. 128. Margaret
Skrovanek: pp. 2; 8-9;
14; 18-19; 46; 89;
122-123; 125; 150.
Christie C. Tito: pp. 4;
30; 31; 36; 37; 99; 152.
Sally Shenk Ullman:
pp. 156; 161.

Other Photographers—
Christopher Barone: pp.
86-87; 102-103. Denny
Gillette: p. 96, bottom
left. Ken Klotz: p. 96, top
left. Daniele Pellegrini,
Photo Researchers, Inc.:
p. 6.

Other Photographs Courtesy of— The Bettman
Archive, N.Y.: pp. 42; 77;
85. Focus on Sports:
p. 50. New Zealand
Tourist Office, N.Y.:
pp. 58-59. Photo
Researchers, Inc.: p. 115.

Illustration Credits

Susan Blubaugh: pp. 3;
14; 25; 47; 48; 63; 76;
101; 111; 119; 157; 162.
Joe Lertola: pp. 5; 8; 16;
20; 26; 27; 28; 39; 49; 51;
55; 56; 57; 61; 71; 73; 94;
98; 104; 116; 136; 146;
148; 158-159, bottom; 160.
Anita Lovitt: pp. 12; 17;
34; 38; 70; 105; 110; 126;
137; 144; 159, top right.
Donna Ruff: pp. 7; 22;
44; 75; 81; 109; 138; 139;
140; 143.

Special Thanks to—
Coronation Cultured
Pearls, Inc., Philadelphia,
Pa.; Dietrich's Meats &
Country Store, Lenharts-
ville, Pa.; Finnaren &
Haley, Inc. Paint Manufac-
turers, Allentown, Pa.;
La Belle Cuisine—Fine
Cookware, Allentown,
Pa.; Richards Jewelers,
Emmaus, Pa.; Ye Olde
Tuxedo Shoppe, Emmaus,
Pa.; YMCA of Bethlehem,
Bethlehem, Pa.

A
Acne, 119-20
Acrodermatitis enteropathica (AE),
85, 115-16
Addiction, nutritional treatment of,
155-63
Air filters, benefits of, 22, 29
Alcohol
effect of, on angina, 17
on blood pressure, 4
on liver, 84
on stomach, 71
toxic effects of, 157
Alcoholism, 157-59
Allergy
arthritis and, 39-40
food, 21-22, 91
Anemia
celiac disease and, 89
use of IUD and, 129
Angina, 1, 14, 17
Anorexia nervosa, 142-43
Antihistamine, vitamin C as, 29
Antioxidants
benefits of for resistance, 27
natural, 55
Appendicitis, 98-100
Arteriolar dilators, 5-6
Arthritis, 33, 34-41. *See also*
Osteoarthritis, Rheumatoid
arthritis, Gout
allergy and, 39-40
drugs for, 40
exercises for, 35, 36-37, 38
psoriatic, benefits of zinc for,
39, 115
treatment of, 34, 40
Aspartame, pros and cons of, 108
Aspirin, 40, 71, 74
asthma attacks due to, 24
benefits of for rheumatoid arthritis,
40
Reye's syndrome and, 153
Asthma
adapting your environment to,
24-26
causes of, 19, 20-22
treatment of, 22-24
Atherosclerosis, 6-14
Autism, nutritional treatment of, 153
B
B vitamins
alcoholism and, 158
cirrhosis and, 85
hearing loss and, 139
importance of to sound mind, 145
sources of, 27
Bedsores, treatment of, 120-21
Beta-carotene, 54, 56
Bile
cholesterol in, 78, 80
gallstone formation and, 78
Binging, 141-42
Biofeedback, benefits of, 23, 146
Birth control pills
cancer and, 64
infertility after use of, 133
Bladder cancer, 66-67
Bleeding, dysfunctional uterine, 128-29
Blindness, hypertension and, 2

Blood pressure, high, steps to lower,
2-3, 4-5
Blood sugar
effect of vitamin E on, 110
regulation of, 104-5
Bowel disease, inflammatory, 90-92
Brain
damage to, from tranquilizers, 160
effects of aging on, 144-45
Breast, self-examination of, 63
Breast cancer, 62-63
Breathing
benefits of exercise for, 29-31
deep, benefits of for angina, 17
Breathing disorders
defense against, 19-31
smoking and, 156
Brewer's yeast, levels of chromium in,
13
Broken hip syndrome, 44-45
Bronchial metaplasia, benefits of
vitamin A for, 57
Bronchitis, 27-28, 29
Bronchospasm, 20-21
Bulimarexia, 142-43
Burns, benefits of vitamin A for, 73
C
Calcium
absorption of, vitamin D and,
45, 98
benefits of, 3-4, 22-23, 98, 152
osteoporosis and, 44
sources of, 4
Cancer, 53-67
bladder, 66-67
breast, 62-63
cervical, 63-65
colorectal, 58-60
endometrial, 64
gastric, formation of, 73
lung, 56-57
nonmelanotic, appearance of, 61
ovarian, 63-65
oxidation and, 55
prostate, 66-67
of sex organs, 56
skin, 60-62
stomach, 65-66
uterine, 63-65
Cataracts, 136-37
Celiac disease, 87-90
Cervical cancer, 63-65
Cervical dysplasia, 64-65
vitamins and, 128
Chemotherapy, benefits of vitamin A
with, 57
Chicken pox, shingles and, 116
Cholesterol, 78-80
effect of vitamin E on, 13
eggs and, 9
heart disease and, 1
Chromium
benefits of for diabetics, 110
effect of on artery plaque, 13
Chronic Obstructive Lung Disease
(C.O.L.D.), 27-29, 31
Circulation, problems with, 1, 16, 110
Cirrhosis, 84-85
Cocaine, 163
Colitis, 90-91

Collagen, importance of vitamins A and C to, 99
Colon cancer, 58-60
Complex partial seizures (CPS), use of choline for, 147
Compression, for treatment of sports injury, 48
Congestion, easing, 31
Congestive heart failure, 2, 5
Continuous passive motion (CPM), 51
Contraceptives, oral. *See* Birth control pills
Copper deficiency, effect of on taste, 140
Cortisone, effect of on lupus, 47
Cramps, menstrual, 124, 126
Crohn's disease, 91-92
Cyclamates, pros and cons of, 108
Cystitis, 100-101

D

Deafness, smoking and, 138
Depression, 151-52
    seasonal, benefits of artificial light for, 150
    severe, definition of, 151
    treatment of, 152
Diabetes, 103-11
    benefits of fiber for, 105, 108-9
    benefits of weight loss for, 109
    circulation problems and, 110
    diet for, 105-11
    heart disease and, 1
    importance of exercise for, 111
    management and prevention of, 104
    nutritional supplements for, 109-11
    types of, 104
Diet
    for alcoholism, 158-59
    for cirrhosis, 85
    cancer and, 54-56, 58, 64-65
    effect of, on atherosclerosis, 8-9, 12
        on gout, 42
    high-fiber, diverticulitis and, 93
    importance of bran in, 93
    kidney stones and, 82-83
    low-purine, guidelines for, 43
    for mind and senses, 135-53
    for quitting smoking, 156-57
    skin health and, 113-21
Dietary fat
    beneficial, 9
    colorectal cancer and, 59
    reducing, 8-9
    high, endometrial cancer and, 64
    low, rheumatoid arthritis and, 39-40
        breast cancer and, 62
Digestive tract
    lower, problems with, 87-101
    upper, problems with, 69-85
Dilators, 5-6
Dimethyl sulfoxide (DMSO), side effects of, 35
Disease, foods that fight, 79
Diuretics, 5
Diverticulitis, 92-94
    cause of, 92
    effect of fiber on, 92, 93
Drugs
    anticholinergic, controversy over, 94
    anticonvulsive, side effects of, 147
    effects of on skin, 119
    prescription, effect of on aging, 144-45
    use of for high blood pressure, 5-6

Dysfunctional uterine bleeding (DUB), 128-29
Dysmenorrhea, treatment of, 126
Dysplasia, cervical, 64
    vitamins and, 65, 128

E

Eicosapentaenoic acid (EPA), benefits of for heart, 9
Elderly, vitamin deficiencies in, 145
Elevation, for treatment of sports injury, 48
Embolism, cerebral, 15
Emotional problems, benefits of diet for, 135-53
Emphysema
    how to ease, 27-28
    problems of gas pains with, 31
Endometrial cancer, 64
Endometriosis, 131-32
Environment
    adapting to asthma attacks, 24-26
    bronchospasm due to, 20-21
    cancer due to, 54
EPA oils, benefits of, 9
Epilepsy, 146-48
    treatment of, 146-47
Epithelial cancer, *See* Skin cancer
Esophageal reflux, 76
Esophagitis, 76-77
Esophagus
    effects of antacids on, 77
    ulceration of, 74
Estrogen replacement therapy (ERT), 64
Exercise(s)
    for angina, 17
    for arthritis, 35, 36-37, 38
    asthma and, 23
    for "blahs," 151
    for breathing, 29-31
    cholesterol levels and, 80
    for cocaine withdrawal, 163
    for diabetics, 111
    after fracture, 51
    for heart, 13-14
    for high blood pressure, 5
    injuries from, 47-51
    nutrition and, benefits of for fertility, 133
    for osteoarthritis, 35
    for premenstrual syndrome, 126
    after stroke, 16
    for strong bones, 45
    for tranquilizer withdrawal, 161
Eye diseases, benefits of nutrition for, 136
Eyes, damage to from superoxides, 136

F

Fat
    amount of in diabetic diet, 109
    colorectal cancer and, 59
    dietary, 8-9
Fertility problems
    causes of, 133
    criterion for, 132
    help for, 132-33
Fever, treatment of in children, 153
Fiber
    action of, 60
    colorectal cancer and, 59-60
    Crohn's disease and, 92
    for diabetics, 105, 108-9
    for diverticulitis, 92
    for hemorrhoids, 95

importance of to kidneys, 83
    sources of, 60, 80, 93-94
    for ulcers, 73, 74
    for weight loss and gallstones, 80
Fibrocystic disease, 62-63
Fish, benefits of in diet, 9, 16, 17
Folate, use of for pneumonia, 27
Folate deficiency
    celiac disease and, 89
    symptoms of, 89
Food(s)
    cancer and, 55
    effect of, on nicotine craving, 157
        on gallstone formation, 80
    to fight disease, 79
    purine-rich, 43
Food allergens
    asthma attacks and, 21-22
    colitis and, 91
    effect of on joints, 39
    most common, 21
    testing for, 21-22
Fractures, treatment of, 50-51
Fructose, pros and cons of, 108

G

Gallstones, 77-81
Gastric cancer, formation of from ulcers, 73
Glaucoma, 136, 137
Glucose tolerance, effect of diuretics on, 5
Glucose tolerance factor (GTF), 110
Glutamine, effect of on alcoholism, 158, 159
Gluten
    effect of on intestine, 88
    psoriasis and, 114
    schizophrenia and, 149-51
    sources of, 88
Gout, 33, 41-43
Gustin, importance of to taste, 140

H

Hearing, 138-39
Hearing loss, benefits of vitamins for, 139
Heart, 1-17
    benefits of exercise for, 13-14
    foods beneficial for, 10
Heart attack, 1, 2, 7
Heart disease, 1
    persons prone to, 1, 14
    vitamin C deficiency and, 12-13
Heart failure, congestive, 2, 5
Heartburn, 74-76
Heberden's nodes, 35
Hemorrhage, cerebral, 15
Hemorrhoidectomy, 96
Hemorrhoids, 94-96
Hernia, hiatal, 74-76
Heroin addiction, vitamin C and, 163
High blood pressure, 1-6
High-fat diet, endometrial cancer and, 64
High-fiber diet, benefits of for diverticulitis, 93
Honey, benefits of for bedsores, 121
Hormones
    effect of on cholesterol in bile, 78
    imbalance in, premenstrual syndrome and, 124
Humidifier, benefits of, 29
Hydrocarbons, levels of in marijuana, 162
Hydrotherapy, benefits of for arthritis, 40